BEHIND THE 'I'M FINE'

THE TRUTH ABOUT MODERN-DAY MASCULINITY

Chris Britton

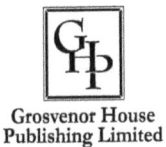

Grosvenor House
Publishing Limited

This book is published by
Grosvenor House Publishing Ltd
Link House
140 The Broadway, Tolworth, Surrey, KT6 7HT.
www.grosvenorhousepublishing.co.uk

A CIP record for this book
is available from the British Library

ISBN 978-1-83615-244-6
eBook ISBN 978-1-83615-245-3

About the Author

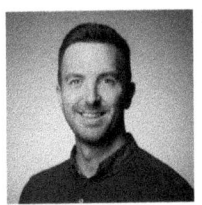 Originally from Northern Ireland but now living in Sussex, UK, Chris is a HR professional with nearly 20 years' experience working across some of the biggest brands in the world, including Vodafone, River Island, Virgin, Samsung, and Reward Gateway. As well as being an author, Chris is a keynote speaker, podcast host, blogger and champion of men's physical and mental health.

Away from work, Chris is a volunteer police officer in Brighton, a football referee in the National League, and a proud father and husband.

You can learn more about Chris on his website: www.chris-britton.com. Get in touch to chat about any events he can support your organisation with.

Connect with Chris across his socials:

- Linked In: https://www.linkedin.com/in/chris-britton-/
- Instagram: @hu_man_up
- TikTok: @hu_manup
- X: chris_britton_
- Bluesky: hu-manup.bsky.social

You can listen to the *Hu-Man Up* podcast on Spotify, YouTube and Apple Podcasts.

Contents

Introduction:
The day that changed it all

I found myself pacing up and down in my lounge, shouting at myself with my internal voice and occasionally letting some of the inner noise out with some heavy sighs. I was so frustrated, I felt I couldn't verbalise how I was feeling; I was so irritated, it made me feel uncomfortable expressing my anxiety. I was desperate for an outlet for my emotions, it was driving me mad!

This was April 2024. I remember it so well – it was early in the morning, it was raining, and it was silent inside my house.

No heartbeat. That is what the sonographer told my wife and I. Our baby had no heartbeat. That feeling of your stomach dropping is quite distinctive; that momentary pause in breathing as you try to absorb exactly what you were just told.

It was our second miscarriage we had suffered that year. The first was in January when the pregnancy was at an earlier stage – just a couple of weeks. We actually talked ourselves into deciding we wouldn't treat it as a miscarriage, rather a late period or a false positive test.

But this second one hurt. Our baby was around 10 weeks, and it had started to form into the shape it was meant to be. We could see it on the scan screen.

It's often said that if you look hard enough, you can find a silver lining in most events. I looked long and hard for that shiny piece of silver, but it was nowhere to be found. All I had was my thoughts, my anger and my questions.

Phew! That was a heavy start to a book. Why on earth have I chosen to start your reading here? Well, I am still searching for that silver lining and, honestly, may never find it.

However, I have been taught some big life lessons; lessons so big that it sparked something inside me to want to share my story, share my lived and learned experiences', and share some of the changes I have made about the way I think. This is all about bringing to the forefront of our conscious thoughts, those things we consider okay to talk about, and open a discussion as to why more stuff needs to be okay to talk about in the future. I approach this specifically from a male perspective. In simple terms, I want men to find the value of being open and honest, no matter the problem or topic.

Although I am not an academic, my views are substantiated by academic research and personal experiences of modern-day men. If you are looking for a book full of hard data and lots of scientific words, then you will get your fill, but this isn't a scholarly textbook. I write from my own lived and learned experiences and by observing the frustrations of other men in the 2020s. I include lots of real-life stories, from real men, who have added their spin on this crazy world and their journey thus far.

Chapter 1:
The Evolution of Masculinity —
from then to now

A so-called crisis in masculinity is not nearly as new as we perhaps think. The concept of masculinity has evolved significantly throughout history, influenced by social, cultural, and political changes. There are well-documented events throughout history as far back as the Ancient Greeks that show being a man and the pressures that go with it, have been a talking point ever since.

Before we take a dive into what is going on in the 21st century, let's take a wander through time to learn about some of the historical evolutions of masculinity, and how that has likely shaped what we see today.

The journey will highlight how definitions of what it means to be a man have been shaped by the needs and values of different societies, often reflecting broader changes in power dynamics, identity, and the role of men in public and private life.

Save our civilisation!

If you know your Greek comedies from your Greek tragedies, then you will already know that the Ancient Greeks had great anxiety over trying to define what it meant to be man in their society, and were obsessed with trying to prove what a 'real' man was.

It was not enough to show that men were physically more powerful than woman; there was a desire to demonstrate, and ultimately prove, that the duty of men was to save civilisation from the rule of women.

A classic example of this is the famous story of Medusa. She was depicted as a gorgon with scary snakes for hair, and anyone who dared to look at her would be immediately turned to stone. The lesser-known part of Medusa's story is how she was punished for being raped and turned into this monster as a way of telling people she had done wrong.

Yet who could stop this stone-turning devil from destroying everyone she looked at?

Enter Perseus, the brave son of Zeus, who quickly catapulted himself into Greek hero status by decapitating the wicked Medusa as she slept. Not enough to conquer the evil serpent lady, Perseus would proudly display Medusa's head as a trophy to signify his strength and victory.

For the Greeks, especially the Spartans, masculinity was synonymous with physical strength, courage, and the ability to fight. The Spartan society, structured around a militaristic way of life, revered warriors as the epitome of manhood. From a young age, Spartan boys were subjected to rigorous training, where they were taught endurance, discipline and combat skills. The ultimate test of a Spartan's worth was his ability to defend his city in battle, with death in combat being the highest honour.

For those who have seen the Gerard Butler movie '300', I know you are now shouting, 'This is Sparta,' in your head. If you have not seen it, I recommend you check it out to see exactly what I mean.

In contrast to Sparta, Athens emphasised a more balanced view of masculinity, combining physical capability with intellectual and philosophical prowess. Athenian men were expected to not only be warriors but also thinkers and philosophers. The pursuit of knowledge, self-control, and rational thought were seen as distinctly masculine traits. Figures like Socrates, Plato and Aristotle embodied this way of thinking, promoting the idea that true manliness included mastery over one's emotions and desires, and a commitment to the pursuit of virtue and wisdom.

All sounds very philosophical, right? Well, you would be right to think that. Yet the fact we are thousands of years on from these men who determined what it meant to be a man, and we still reference and sometimes revere them, tells you everything you need to know about their power and influence. It also tells you that in all that time, we have failed to define masculinity in any other way than they did. There are lots of examples of evolution all over the place. We are far more sophisticated in many ways, but updating our view of what it means to be a man? Not so much.

Greek masculinity was also characterised by the importance of relationships between men, particularly in the context of the symposium (a social gathering for men) and the gymnasium (a space for physical exercise and intellectual discussion). These environments reinforced the masculine principles of camaraderie, loyalty, and mentorship.

In some Greek cities, such as Athens, pederasty (a socially acknowledged relationship between an adult male and a younger male) was an accepted and even idealised practice, believed to help the younger to grow into a 'full man' by acquiring the knowledge and virtues of the elder. This could be some of the earliest documented mentoring relationships. The relationships got so deep, they often turned sexual.

Ancient Greek men certainly got around; they slept with their wives, slaves and young protégés. A real powerplay of sexual dominance.

Be Brave, Be Moral, Be Roman!

As the Greek way of life declined, the Roman Republic rose to prominence, carrying forward and transforming many Greek ideals of masculinity. The Roman concept of masculinity, or *virtus*, was deeply intertwined with the notions of strength, honour, and duty to the state.

The term *virtus* derives from *vir*, meaning man. It encapsulated a range of qualities expected of Roman men: bravery in battle, moral integrity, and unwavering commitment to Rome. Unlike the Greeks who balanced the physical with the intellectual, Roman masculinity was singularly focused on action and public service. A Roman man's worth was often measured by his achievements in war and his contributions to the political life of the Republic. The Roman paterfamilias (head of the household) also exemplified masculine authority, holding absolute power over his family and slaves.

This part of history still fascinates us today. I have lost count of the number of documentaries I have seen on the Romans, all telling a similar tale – of family life, complete devotion to the state, innovation, and world domination.

The shift from philosopher to warrior started us on a journey to defining modern-day masculinity, and many misconceptions with it can be attributed to our toga-wearing ancestors.

Ever wondered from where the notion that 'real men do not cry' came? In my opinion, it could be traced back to the Romans and the importance society placed on remaining nonplussed in the face of adversity.

Stoic teachings emphasised self-control, rationality, and emotional resilience – qualities that became central to the Roman male identity. A Roman man was expected to maintain composure, to prioritise reason over passion, and to embody the virtues of endurance and temperance.

As the Empire expanded, so did the demands of its men. Masculinity began to be associated with Imperial authority and dominance. Emperors like Augustus cultivated a public image of idealised masculinity, combining military success with moral and familial virtues.

But even back then, the public image of such men did not always tally with what was happening behind closed doors. As the Roman Empire continued to grow, the traditional outwardly facing characteristics of masculinity started to erode, replaced by lavish decadence and greed. This, as is well documented, did not end well for the Romans!

The Rise of Religion

The fall of the Roman Empire and the rise of Christianity brought about significant changes to the concept of masculinity. During the Medieval period, masculinity became intertwined with the ideals of chivalry and Christian virtue, reflecting the social and religious transformations of the time.

In Medieval Europe, the figure of the knight came to represent the pinnacle of manliness. Things like the chivalric code, which governed the behaviour of knights, emphasised martial skill, honour, and loyalty, and love was formed and this quickly translated into followers. A knight was expected to be a formidable warrior, but also to protect the weak, and uphold justice. This duality–strength combined with moral integrity–became the hallmark of medieval masculinity.

Christianity introduced new dimensions to the concept of manhood. The Christian view of masculinity emphasised humility, piety, and self-sacrifice. The figure of Christ, who embodied these virtues, became a model for Christian men. Monasticism, which required vows of celibacy, poverty, and obedience, offered an alternative form of masculinity that rejected the traditional markers of male status, such as wealth, power, and sexual prowess. This period also saw the veneration of saints, many of whom were men who had demonstrated extraordinary faith and moral fortitude.

But of course, like many periods in history, differing opinions led to clashes and all-out war. Medieval masculinity was marked by a tension between the violent warrior ethos of the knight and the peaceful, spiritual ideals of Christianity. These juxtaposed viewpoints often created conflicts in the expectations placed on men, particularly those in positions of power, who were expected to lead both in battle and in moral guidance. The Crusades, for instance, were seen as a way to reconcile these competing perspectives, with knights framing their military exploits as acts of piety and service to God.

In modern times, there is a school of thought that suggests the relevant downfall of religion, with society instead of becoming much more secular, has played a role in shaping masculinity. Whatever your personal stance on religion, it is difficult to dispute that religion does offer some form of moral guardrails for humanity.

Rightly or wrongly, most religions offer a prescribed way of behaving, interacting, relationship management and socialisation. Of course, you do not need to be religious to form your own moral compass but if you are a follower of religion and do not follow the word of whichever God you worship, then you open yourself up to your own punishment. The risk of burning in hell, purgatory, or never seeing your loved ones again in heaven, certainly can work to keep people in check and to make what they perceive as the right decisions.

We should all be more like Da Vinci!

The Renaissance period and the philosophical movement known as the Enlightenment witnessed further shifts in the concept of masculinity, as new ideas about individuality, reason, and society began to take hold.

The Renaissance mindset of the *uomo universale* (universal man) reflected a new vision of masculinity, combining physical, intellectual, and artistic prowess. Renaissance thinkers like Leonardo da Vinci and Michelangelo embodied this thinking, excelling in multiple disciplines and emphasising the importance of cultivating all aspects of their potential. This period saw a renewed interest in the classical ways of thinking of Greece and Rome, but with a greater emphasis on individual achievement and expression.

The phrase 'Renaissance Man' is still used today. The 1994 movie of the same name sees actor Danny DeVito play the role of a down-and-out salesman taking on the challenge of teaching literacy to a group of disinterested army students. He struggles at first, but after introducing them to the wonders of Shakespeare, the students' views are transformed. This feel-good comedy aims to show how opening one's mind to different things and new perspectives can have a positive impact on how you think and feel, unlocking a potential you might not know you have. Maybe something we should all try in our modern, increasingly divisive world.

Philosophers like John Locke further transformed the notion of masculinity, placing a premium on reason, education, and civic responsibility. If that name sounds familiar, it is likely you are a fan of the hit TV show *Lost*. That John Locke was certain he had been chosen by the Island to serve a purpose and went on a journey of self-discovery about who he was and what he stood for. I digress. Locke and fellow philosopher Jean-Jacques Rousseau argued that men were naturally rational beings, and that their primary role was to contribute to the betterment of society through reasoned debate and action. The ideal man was no longer just a warrior or a saint, but a rational, educated citizen who could participate in the governance of society.

The Enlightenment movement also saw the emergence of a new domestic way of thinking about the role of a man. Men were increasingly expected to not only be public figures, but also moral and responsible heads of households. The family became a microcosm of the state, with the father as the ruler who exercised authority with wisdom and justice. Sound familiar? Indeed, this shift laid the groundwork for the modern concept of the nuclear family, where masculinity was defined, in part, by the man's ability to provide for and protect his family.

Industry, War and Feminism

The 19th and 20th centuries brought about significant challenges to traditional notions of masculinity, as industrialisation, war and social change reshaped the world. All significant events in their own right, right up to the 21st century these generational changes shaped how we define masculinity.

The Industrial Revolution fundamentally altered the structure of society, leading to the rise of the urban working class and the middle-class view of the breadwinner. Men's identities became increasingly tied to their role as providers, with masculinity being measured by an ability to earn a living and support a family. This period also saw the emergence of the 'self-made man', a belief that celebrated individual success and economic independence.

The two world wars of the 20th century had a profound impact on masculinity. The mass mobilisation of men for combat reinforced traditional masculine ideals of bravery and sacrifice, while also exposing the fragility and destructiveness of these ways of thinking. The trauma of war led to widespread questioning of the value of the warrior view, with many men returning from the front lines physically and psychologically scarred.

They called it shell shock back then; we now commonly refer to it as post-traumatic stress disorder (PTSD). Research into this psychological condition has evolved rapidly in modern times as we begin to understand much more about the brain, and how it is impacted by experiences – both physically (how the actual structure of the brain alters due to trauma), and emotionally (how our thoughts and actions are triggered by certain stimuli).

The evolution of science-based studies looking at our emotions and, more broadly, mental health, have changed how we talk and empathise with conditions like PTSD. But during the immediate post-war period, however, the approach would have been very different story. Those returning from war with PTSD (almost exclusively men) would have been assessed using a rigid scale of emotions, from 'feeling a bit sad' through to 'completely mad'. With little or no treatment available and a complete lack of understanding about what these men were experiencing, society locked them away, forgot all about them, or simply stoked the fires with the offhand comment, 'man up'. This mindset continues even today with many veterans of war or conflict never speaking of their experiences and letting it consume them.

Notwithstanding the immediate aftermath of World War One and World War Two the post-war periods saw a crisis of masculinity, as traditional roles were increasingly called into question by social changes, including the Feminist Movement.

The late 20th and early 21st centuries have witnessed the emergence of new, more diverse understandings of the meaning and role of a man. The feminist and LGBTQIA+ movements have challenged traditional gender roles, leading to greater acceptance of alternative forms of masculinity that reject rigid stereotypes.

The rise of feminism, with the ultimate goal of creating economic independence for women, has fundamentally changed the landscape we are all now a part of. The gender pay gap is still real and there is a long way to go, but we should celebrate the success of closing that gap over the past few decades, while also being able to discuss how it has reshaped the role of men in our society.

Today, masculinity is increasingly seen as a spectrum, with room for emotional expression, vulnerability, and a rejection of toxic behaviours. The concept of 'toxic masculinity' has gained traction, highlighting the negative side of what it means to be a man today, and recently has led to a surge in the desire to turn 'toxic' into 'positive' masculinity.

The Quest for Positive Masculinity Has Created an Identity Crisis

All right, that is the end of our history lesson.

So, what does it mean to be a man in the 21st century?

Picture the scene: generation after generation of males being told that being a man means all those things we just talked about: strength, courage, control, being the provider; emotionless, stiff upper lip, 'man up'.

Then, in just one generation, everything that has been indoctrinated in the physical and social DNA of males is now seen as toxic. We are challenging the role of men in our society for all the right reasons: equality, equity, fairness. But that does not change the fact that everything you thought you knew about yourself–who you stand for, and your place in the world–is now under attack.

What impact is that having on men right now?

Well, the sad truth is, being a man, especially a young man (I am talking mid-teens through to mid-twenties), is now a confusing place. The pandemic changed a lot of things in our lives including how we work, but let's not forget it also had a profound impact on our relationships and our ability to form new ones. However, even if we took out the impact that the pandemic had on the most formative years of those young men, the march for female equality has absolutely had an unintentional consequence. It has left men with an identity crisis which is fuelling a generation of anger, resentment, mental health breakdowns, frustration, mixed messaging and polarising behaviour.

What it means to be a man is now unclear. A once rigid and clearly marked space in society has been demolished. In times of uncertainty and complexity, human beings try to make things simple. So, let's seek out the easiest path; let me find voices who speak to me in a language I understand.

Right now, young men are being pushed to one of two sides of the masculinity debate.

On one side, option A, is the positive masculinity camp. This is all about men displaying behaviours more typically associated with femininity: showing empathy, expressing emotions, being kind, talking about feelings, etcetera. There is absolutely nothing wrong with men leaning more towards this side of the debate, indeed the world would be a better place if we were all a little kinder and a little more empathetic.

However, one of the issues with positive masculinity is how it is currently marketed. It is normally coming from angle of telling men off rather than helping men understand what great things they can bring to the conversation. In simple terms (and I am paraphrasing here slightly), the confusing rationale for positive masculinity can be summed up by saying: be less like a man and more like a woman.

So, what about option B?

Option B is those people arguing for a time machine to take us back a few generations. Let's call it 'conversative' masculinity. This is the camp that would rather the evolution of masculinity didn't happen at all, and in fact think that men should remain 'typical; men and women should remain 'typical' women. This conversative view of the world can be summed up like this: men have spent millennia doing what men do, why on earth should we change it now? Men should be strong, dominant, emotionless, and assert themselves on the world and those within it.

If you are a young man, and you are given option A (be less man, be more woman) or option B (do what you have always done and be the stronger sex), realistically, to which are you going to subscribe?

The answer to that question will split opinion, and it is very complex. A lot of factors will come into play, some of which I am going to dig into throughout this book. Things like role models, socioeconomic background, access to and use of social media, culture, race, financial health, family unit, neurodiversity, and even the careers that men have, all play a part in how men find their purpose and sense of identity. Historically, all those factors existed and still played a part in determining the 'type' of man someone would turn out to be. But there was always a default position to fall back on and a generally accepted view of what being a man really meant.

But now?

As I write this book in 2024, I believe only having those two viable options is dangerous, and we must work to find a middle ground between option A and B. We must produce an option C that gives men an identity without slowing down the amazing progress being made in relation to unrepresented inclusion and equality.

We have greatly underestimated the impact of the evolutionary change in how men behave and interact in our world, and what you will see throughout the book are facts, stories and suggested solutions for creating option C.

I heard a quote recently from the wonderfully outspoken, yet rational, Steven Bartlett. Steven is an entrepreneur, famous for his role on hit BBC business investment show *Dragons' Den*. But first and foremost, Steven is a successful businessman who spends time investing in the betterment of work and treating people fairly, using his platform to educate society by interviewing business leaders and thought leaders on his successful podcast *Diary of a CEO*. On one particular episode, Steven's words resonated with me:

> 'We have spent a long time now calling men out for their behaviour. To really change, it is time we start calling men back in.'

This resonated with me because I am a believer that to flourish, we need to work together rather than against each other.

To really move society forward, all men must join the same journey. We do not need to push men down to lift anyone else up; society will only reach its full potential when *all* sides are elevated. There is space for everyone. We need men to be part of the inclusion agenda and to feel like they have a purpose.

A big part of the creation of option C is to talk about the things men typically don't talk about. We need guys to feel comfortable in their skin, be aware of their behaviours, acknowledge their feelings, and be a positive contributor to our world.

So, let's begin the journey together. Join me as we explore lots of different areas we need to talk about openly and honestly, so we can work towards addressing the masculinity crisis emerging today.

Chapter 2:
Men's Health Uncovered

In recent decades, the subject of men's health has garnered increased attention, as alarming statistics reveal the silent crisis unfolding across the Western world. The intersection of physical and mental health challenges among men paints a concerning picture, a picture often overshadowed by societal norms, stigma, fear, and inadequate approaches by healthcare professionals. This chapter delves into the statistics surrounding men's physical and mental health, uncovering the trends and disparities, and highlighting the urgent need for action.

The old-fashioned notion of masculinity, often associated with self-reliance, stoicism, and physical strength, can deter men from seeking medical help or acknowledging their mental health struggles.

The Brain is Often Louder than the Beating Heart

While physical health concerns are more widely recognised, mental health issues among men are equally pressing but far less discussed. Depression, anxiety and suicide are major threats men face, often in silence due to cultural and societal expectations and misguided feelings of shame and embarrassment.

Men are significantly less likely than women to seek help for mental health problems. For example, statistics from Substance Abuse and Mental Health Services Administration (SAMHSA) in the USA, indicate that men account for only 36% of all mental health therapy clients.[1]

One of the most alarming statistics is the suicide rate among men. The World Health Organisation (WHO) reported that in countries such as the United States, the United Kingdom, Australia and Canada, men are three–four times more likely to die by suicide than women.[2] In the UK, according to the National Health Service (NHS) suicide is the biggest killer amongst men under the age of 50.[3]

This is despite all the effort and spotlight that has been shone on men's mental health in the past 10 years or so; this is despite the constant calls for improvement to mental health services more broadly, this is despite

---

1 Substance Abuse and Mental Health Services Administration. (2021). *Behavioural Health Equity Barometer*. Rockville, MD: SAMHSA

2 World Health Organization. (2021). *Suicide Worldwide in 2021: Global Health Estimates*. Available at: https://www.who.int [Accessed 30th August 2024].

3 Sutherland, R. (2018). *NHS England-Tackling the root causes of suicide*. (online) Available at https://www.england.nhs.uk/blog/tackling-the-root-causes-of-suicide/[Accessed 20th September 2024].

men being far more aware of these statistics than perhaps at any other time in our history.

But it is not working. The suicide statistics in particular continue on a worryingly upward trend.

As a teenager growing up in Northern Ireland, I fell into the same trap that I suspect a lot of young men do. I got swept up in the pretence of what I thought a man should be, likely influenced heavily by those male role models around me. I did not talk openly about how I felt, and I very rarely showed my true emotions.

As I moved into life as an adult, attending university in Brighton and studying criminology and psychology, my experience of growing up had made me guarded, unwilling to let people get too close to me. Whenever anyone asked how I was, I'd always reply, 'Fine thanks,' irrespective of the truth.

The truth of the matter was that underneath my emotionless exterior, I was struggling with finding my way in the world. I had friends, I had a family, I had a good job. On the face of it, what did I have to complain about?

It took me a while before realising something was not right and I gathered the courage to visit a doctor. Not just any doctor, a male one, someone I was hoping I could relate to or would empathise with me. The actual outcome of my first visit to the GP to talk about how I felt left me feeling more confused than ever. I felt I was not taken seriously:

"Fill in this form," said the GP without really engaging in a conversation. "We cannot do anything until you fill this in. But you cannot do it now as I am busy, so you will need to make another appointment to come back."

I was persistent, and I pushed to be seen again quickly with my completed form. However, I can understand why some men would be affected by that negative experience and never seek help again. We know that men don't seek help as much as women, so when a male musters up the courage to talk, it's imperative the medical professional is willing to listen.

The cultural stigma of not wanting to be seen as vulnerable, and the lack of adequate support when a man does ask for help, no doubt leads to a significant under reporting of mental health issues among men.

Here for a Good Time, Not a Long Time

Historically, men have had shorter life expectancies than women, and this trend continues to persist across most Western countries. For instance, in the US, the average life expectancy for men is approximately 76 years, compared to 81 years for women.[4] Similar

4 Center for Disease Control and Prevention. (2022). *Leading Causes of Death, All Men*. Available at: https://www.cdc.gov [Accessed 30th October 2024]

patterns are observed in other Western nations, with women consistently outliving men by 4–7 years.[5]

The leading causes of death among men also include heart disease, cancer, unintentional injuries, chronic lower respiratory diseases, and stroke. Cardiovascular disease remains the most significant contributor, accounting for nearly one in four male deaths. Men are less likely than women to visit a doctor regularly, even when experiencing symptoms of illness. They are also less likely to adhere to prescribed treatment, which can lead to worsening health.

Hands up any guy reading this who has ever been in pain but not visited a doctor? Or had medication prescribed to them, and then just not taken it? Yeah, me too.

The nonchalant attitude of 'I'm fine' is a pretty dangerous one, physically and mentally.

The waiting lists for things like Cognitive Behaviour Therapy (CBT) or other talking therapies in the UK are long; Unsurprising given what we know about the general state of mental health support in the western world.

The GP I visited offered to refer me and add me to the waiting list, but I turned him down. The thought of having to wait for months to be seen didn't appeal to

---

5 World Health Organisation (WHO). (2023). *World Health Statistics 2023*. Geneva: WHO

me at all. So, I pushed for medication; I wanted an instant fix.

To his credit, the GP advised against it and said we should try different things first like exercise, getting fresh air, talking to family and friends. These are all tried, tested and valid preventative measures for things like anxiety and depression. But maybe because I am just impatient (or maybe because I am a man), I insisted I wanted the medication, he ultimately agreed and started me off on a small dose.

So, off I went to the pharmacy around the corner with my prescription for Citalopram (one of the various brands of medication that are used to help stabilise moods). As I waited in the pharmacy, with other people collecting their medication, I could not help but wonder if I looked depressed to them.

Did I look sad? Was the pharmacist surprised by who was handing over the prescription? Did the people collecting their own medication look at me and think there is something wrong with him? Truthfully, I just wanted to grab my medication and get out of there as quickly as possible. So, with my head bowed, I spoke quietly to confirm my name and address, grabbed the bag and exited the pharmacy, hoping I had managed to stay under the radar.

Walking quickly home, I had a lot of different emotions running through my head—a little bit of embarrassment and definitely some shame—but I also felt positive that my instant remedy to my feelings and emotions was in my hands, in the form of this tiny box of pills.

For anyone reading this who has taken antidepressants, you will know the spiel that the doctor gives you: 'It's going to get worse before it gets better. The medication takes time to work through your system, and your body will need time to adjust to the new chemicals going to work on your thoughts and feelings.'

My view? 'Nah, it will be fine.'

Turns out, the medical professionals do know what they are talking about; certainly, more than the jumbled thoughts of a 24-year-old who wanted a miracle cure. The first few weeks of taking antidepressants is like riding an emotional rollercoaster: the waves of energy that run through your body for no random reason, the leg twitches, the sharp inhaling of air out of nowhere. But after a few weeks, that does simmer down and things start to settle a little.

All good, right?

Well, my impatient and stubborn brain wasn't happy with how it was making me feel and I talked myself into thinking that I did not need the medication. I decided it was pointless, and it was making me worse rather than better. So, I stopped without consulting the GP. There was no weaning off period, and, in the interests of complete transparency, it made me feel awful.

The stats which show that men live less than women, in my opinion one of those reasons is because men sometimes ignore professional medical advice. I had medication proven to treat the symptoms of the ailment from which I was suffering; I had worked up the courage to go to the GP and fight for the medicine rather than join an endless queue of people on a growing waiting list, and I braved the pharmacy and rode out the first few weeks of my body adjusting.

Then I just decided I knew better and stopped without consulting a medical professional. This is a cautionary tale for anyone reading this, but especially men. The medical folks know more than you do and certainly know more than Dr Google. If someone who is qualified, regulated and experienced suggests a treatment plan (medication-based or otherwise), it is probably worth adhering to and letting it run its course, rather than trying to do it your way....

On the waiting list point, there are lots of reasons why the lists are getting bigger and longer. Successive governments in the UK have promised more funding and a fresh approach to try and tackle this growing problem and that work continues. The simple truth is that demand is outstripping supply. A key reason why prevention must be a better option than cure.

The Health and Safety Executive (HSE) reports that the vast majority of injuries and/or deaths in the workplace come from men.[6] With a figure as high as 95%, this is a reflection of the type of work that men historically have taken on and some of the risks involved. I would also throw into the mix that perhaps us guys are less likely to pay close attention to health and safety in the workplace, and maybe a little bit of showboating or ego-massaging could factor into the injuries suffered on the job. I certainly have ignored workplace guidance about standing on ladders, wedging doors open or not using a microwave in the office kitchen.

Furthermore, men are more likely than women to engage in behaviours that increase their risk of premature death, such as smoking, excessive alcohol consumption, and neglecting regular health check-ups. In fact, men are almost three times more likely to become dependent on alcohol and are more likely to report regular use of drugs (recreational or otherwise) than women.

Does it Matter Where you are From?

I'd love to say the answer to this question is no. But sadly, socioeconomic status plays a critical role in the

---

6 Health and Safety Executive. (2024). *Fatal injuries arising from accidents at work in Great Britain*. Available at https://www.hse.gov.uk/statistics/gender/index.htm [Accessed 30th October 2024]

health outcomes of men. In his book, *The Health Gap*, Professor Sir Michael Marmot talks about how men in lower income brackets often have less access to quality healthcare and less healthcare awareness in general. Couple those things with higher exposure to risk factors like poor diet, hazardous work environments, and chronic stress, and you can see why being a guy from a disadvantaged background could have a negative impact on your health and wellbeing.

Unemployment is also a significant factor that disproportionately affects men, particularly during economic downturns. In 2010, David Wilkins published a piece of research in the Men's Health Forum which highlights why historic views of masculinity can lead to more issues for men over women. He talks about the roles that men have in the workplace and how just by the way society is constructed (i.e. men typically are paid more and have always been expected to the breadwinner) then the psychological toll of job loss or financial instability is magnified.[7] It can dial up mental health issues, leading to a vicious cycle of deteriorating physical and mental wellbeing.

---

7 Wilkins, D. (2010). *Untold problems A review of the essential issues in the mental health of men and boys. Published by* Men's Health Forum. Available at: https://www.menshealthforum.org.uk/sites/default/files/pdf/untold_problems.pdf.

2024 research from employee engagement company Reward Gateway showed that employed people across the UK rated their financial wellbeing as their biggest concern in the last two years.[8] If you are guy, not working or on a low income and wondering how on earth you are going to meet the demands of bills, rent, healthcare costs etc., then you can see why socioeconomic status is a huge variable in relation to one's state of mind and overall health. Especially when combined with the other factors we have explored already.

In addition to this, the Centre of Disease Control and Prevention in the USA show that men in economically disadvantaged groups are more likely to engage in harmful behaviours, such as smoking and substance abuse,[9] further contributing to poor health outcomes. These behaviours are often coping mechanisms for stress but ultimately lead to higher rates of chronic disease and early death. 'A perfect storm' comes to mind.

8 Reward Gateway. (2024). *The HR Priority Report 2024.* Available at: https://www.rewardgateway.com/uk/resource/the-hr-priority-report-2024 [Accessed 24 November 2024]

9 Centre for Disease Control and Prevention. (2022). *Leading Causes of Death, All Men.* Available at: https://www.cdc.gov [Accessed 30th October 2024]

Does it Matter What your Job is?

I just explored how socioeconomic status can have an impact on the outcomes of health amongst unemployed males. But what about guys who do paid work? Are there any links between the job that someone does and the risk to their health – physical or mental?

While more research needs to be carried out to really shine a light on this, there are emerging trends on certain occupations being at higher risk of death. Perhaps unsurprisingly, dangerous roles involving machinery, lots of driving, and the military would be near the top of the list.

But can we see any links between job roles and suicide rates? The Office for National Statistics (ONS) in the UK published data in May 2024 showing suicide rates across England and Wales between 2020–2022.[10]

For men aged between 20–64, the research shows a clear leader in terms of which job group has the highest suicide rate: skilled trade/construction.

In the UK, in 2024 a campaign was launched called the Lost City[11] to remember the 7000 construction

---

10 GOV.UK. *Statistical commentary: suicide prevention profile, May 2024 update.* Available at: https://www.gov.uk/government/statistics/suicide-prevention-profile-updates/statistical-commentary-suicide-prevention-profile-may-2024-update.

11 The Lost City. (2024). *The Lost City.* Available at: https://www.thelostcity.org/

workers who committed suicide in the last 10 years. To show the scale of that, the campaign talks about the city of the equivalent size of Cardiff not being built due to the mental health crisis in the construction industry, with as many as two tradespeople a day taking their own lives.

Continuing down the statistics rabbit hole, the ONS data shows that the suicide rate in construction is four times the national average, and UK tradespeople are 26% more likely than other workers to experience mental ill health.

These shocking statistics clearly beg the question, why?

We know that mental health funding in the western world is in short supply, and we know that despite whatever offer of help is available, men are less likely to engage. But what is it about a specific industry like construction that adds so much additional pressure to the lives of those working in it? It really links back into a lot of the themes we have already discussed and will be discussing later, such as, loneliness, financial pressure, the notion of masculinity, and a lack of confidence in talking about feelings and emotions.

On The Tools, the UK's largest tradespeople community, works to amplify voices and provide support and resources to the lives of workers. They say that as many as 96% of tradespeople work on their own[12], isolated in the workplace. This might be your reality, but if it is not, could you imagine working on your own for prolonged periods of time? Some people might say, yes please, sign me up! But the truth is, isolation heightens the risk of developing poor mental health.

How about the financial pressures? On The Tools state that 65% of tradespeople suffer financial stress, often exacerbated by inconsistent payments. They also report only 32% of workers have access to counselling, with many unaware of available resources and support systems.

I am sure there are lots of workers in different industries who, upon reading this, will think they face similar issues. My take on the stats is that this is a male-dominated industry, with access to heavy machinery or tools which can (intentionally or otherwise) inflict harm easily, and all of those factors are intersecting at the same time.

If you were wondering about your own profession, then just for completeness, in October 2024 the *HR Review* magazine published the 10 most stressful

---

12 Dowd, L. (2024). *Construction workers four times more likely to die by suicide as 7,000 lives lost, report says*. Sky News. Available at: https://news.sky.com/story/construction-workers-four-times-more-likely-to-die-by-suicide-as-7-000-lives-lost-report-says-13272758.

professions in the UK.[13] The data is based on reported numbers of people in those professions who have recorded some form of mental ill health.

Interestingly, construction and tradespeople do not appear on this list.

What does that tell me? I don't think you have to leap too far to see that jobs that are primarily done by men who do not report or talk about their feelings are the ones with final and sad endings. Just because things go unreported, does not mean there is not a problem bubbling beneath the surface. The shocking ONS statistics are a grim reminder of what happens when men don't talk. We need to get guys talking before it is too late.

Don't Forget About Me!

In the next chapter, I will explore the importance of community amongst men. It's an area often taken for granted but has a huge role to play if we are to truly get to the bottom of how we solve the issues with masculinity.

---

13 HR Review. (2024). *Most Stressful Jobs in the UK Revealed.* Available at: https://hrreview.co.uk/hr-news/wellbeing-news/most-stressful-jobs-in-the-uk-revealed/377020 [Accessed 20th September 2024].

Loneliness and social isolation are growing concerns, particularly among older men. As men age, they often experience a decline in social networks due to retirement, the death of peers, or divorce. In the UK, 1.26 million men over the age of 65 live alone. This number is higher in women, but unlike women, who tend to maintain more robust social connections throughout their lives, men are more susceptible to becoming socially isolated, which can have severe implications for both physical and mental health.[14]

Research has shown that social isolation increases the risk of mortality, with some studies suggesting that its impact is comparable to smoking or obesity. The National Institute for Ageing report that men who are socially isolated are at a higher risk of developing mental health issues such as depression and anxiety, and they are also more likely to engage in harmful behaviours like excessive drinking or drug taking.[15]

I was born in 1987 (you can do the math as to how old I am). Growing up, I was never the most popular

---

14 Beach, B. and Bamford, S.-M. (2018). *Isolation: The emerging crisis for older men A report exploring experiences of social isolation and loneliness among older men in England*. Available at: https://ilcuk.org.uk/wp-content/uploads/2018/10/Loneliness-in-older-men-report.pdf. [Accessed 30th August 2024].

15 National Institute on Aging. (2020). *Social Isolation, Loneliness and Health*. Bethesda, MD: National Institute on Aging. Available at: https://www.nia.nih.gov [Accessed 30th August 2024].

kid, but I did flip between friendship groups. I was cool but I was not cool enough for some; I wasn't so amazing at sports that I could play in the A team, but I was good enough for the B side. I had lots of acquaintances rather than true friends, though I did have a small inner circle of friends with whom I loved hanging out.

As I got older, and especially at university, my friendship group burgeoned. I made many friends for life there, pushed together as we were by the roommate lottery. Though a few people have come and gone over the years from that group, the majority remain.

My reputation among my core friendship groups has always been that I rarely socialise. In a way, I prefer my own company. But it did also bother me a little (and still does) why I never really saw myself as a sociable person. Up until I met my wife, there was a real risk that I would grow old alone, as I really never found the confidence to go into a social setting and chat to girls. In truth, it riddled me with anxiety, and if it wasn't for the wonders of dating apps, where I could express my interest in someone and get the initial formalities out of the way digitally, I might well have never found a partner.

I am less concerned about the future and growing old on my own now. But my friendship group from university? Well, I see them less and less. One thing I have always prided myself on is being the voice of reason, the one who would drop everything to help people I care about. I hope I am still that person and that my university friends know that, despite not seeing each other very often now.

Boys are typically rubbish at checking in on their mates, and I am no exception. It's easy to see how male friendships drift over time and people lose contact. Why do men struggle to remain connected?

It could be an emotional intelligence thing. But I think at the heart of it is that men often feel nervous asking how people are. We would not be entirely comfortable if the response was, 'I'm not OK,' as we would instinctively try to fix the problem without truly listening.

A call to action here if you are a guy reading this: you now know that the isolation statistics aren't favourable for men, especially as we get older, and all the inherent problems that creates. So, if you have a mate that you keep meaning to check in on, stop reading, pick up your phone and call them or WhatsApp right now. I can wait...

Welcome back. That was not too difficult, right? Reconnect with your male friends; don't become a future statistic.

So Now we Know, So What?

Addressing the crisis in men's physical and mental health requires a carefully considered and thoughtful reimagining. We need to continue with our public health initiatives that focus on increasing awareness, reducing stigma, and promoting health-seeking behaviours among men. Healthcare systems must adapt to better meet the needs of men, particularly in terms of mental health support and preventive care.

Easy right? Not so. A lot of that has already been done: money spent, resources used, and conversations had. So, what needs to change?

Education is key to changing the narrative around masculinity and health. Campaigns that encourage men and boys to talk about their health, both physical and mental, and to seek help when needed, can have a profound impact. Additionally, integrating mental health services into primary care settings can make it easier for men to access the support they need without the added stigma of seeking specialised care.

I argue that the workplace needs to do more, because interventions can also play a crucial role. Employers should not only promote mental health awareness, provide access to counselling services, and create a work environment that supports health and wellbeing, but should also help to connect men in safe spaces to allow open dialogue about behaviour, identity, men's health and more. Also, addressing the unique challenges faced by men in different socioeconomic groups is essential for reducing physical and mental health disparities.

More work also needs to be done to dispel the myths of fatherhood and create more support and openness around the difficulties of being a dad, balancing that with work and all the stereotypical views of being a man that go with it.

So-called taboo topics need to be binned. Men suffer from male-specific issues and that is absolutely OK! The more we talk about things like prostate and testicular cancers, erectile dysfunction, miscarriage through a dad's eyes, the impact of hair loss, body image and lots of others, the better. An uncomfortable conversation is usually worth having.

For those men, in those industries or jobs that typically work alone (I am talking about sole traders etc.) then this responsibility of connection and safe spaces falls on society to do more.

On the topic of society, collectively we need to get a grip on our communities and show young men that their behaviour has a huge impact on not only their lives but those around them. We need to do better at showing young men that their choices have consequences – unintended or otherwise.

Finally, there is a need for more research focused specifically on men's health. Understanding the gender-specific factors that contribute to health outcomes will allow for more targeted and effective interventions going forward. It is my hope that the topics I discuss in this book will spark conversations between men, and that the willingness to discuss previously difficult or sensitive topics goes some way to making a difference.

The statistics surrounding men's physical and mental health highlights a crisis that is profound but still largely hidden. Men are at higher risk of a range of physical and mental health issues, yet they are less likely to seek help or engage in preventive behaviours. By acknowledging the unique challenges that men face and taking steps to address them, society can begin to turn the tide on this silent crisis, improving the health and wellbeing of millions of men across the world.

Understanding the 'Whys' of the Men's Health Challenge

A key theme of this book, as you will discover, are the real-life stories, the sharing of expertise and experiences of modern-day men. One such expert is Joe Gaunt, a stage one health psychologist and doctoral researcher. Joe is also the founder and CEO of Zeno Health Group and co-founder and CEO of men's health brand Unify.

The following story is recounted in Joe's own words.

Joe's Story

The landscape for men in the modern age has never looked more challenging.

All research and evidence point to the consistent facts that across the globe, men live shorter lives, consistently experiencing lower quality of life (or 'health span') within those years.

At the two extreme ends of the scale, highly male-dominant environments still live in the man-up-I'm-fine-be-tough-and-don't-show-weakness mentality. At the opposite end, men's roles have never felt more confusing to many who are used to or seek more traditional roles of providing for family or being chivalrous.

It is perhaps no wonder, then, that four out of five suicides are men, and the numbers are increasing over time.

As a trained psychologist, I would always look to a biopsychosocial (Engel, 1980) framework (including socioeconomics) as a determinant of health and life status for each individual and group. There are then specific psychological and psychosocial drivers that shape some of the stats and health outcomes for men.[16]

A known health paradox between men and women is that women 'need' or attend more health services than men and live longer.

---

16 Engel GL. (1980) *The clinical application of the biopsychosocial model.* Am J Psychiatry.137(5):535-44.

Applying a degree of common sense, the important element here we can interpret is that women generally are more comfortable in both verbalising issues and showing vulnerability informally to friends and family. Women are also more likely to be comfortable seeking the professional help they need, which in turn gives them targeted support.

Unfortunately, this is not the case for men. Men are much more likely to mask feelings from friends and family because they feel they are expected to be 'the strong one'. Men in general also tend to lean towards outcome-focused problem-solving and may not value or see the relevance of simply talking about things.

So, the issues remain. Men often feel trapped and seek escape as a means of coping. Consequently, men are more likely to engage in what would be termed 'negative' coping behaviours such as drinking alcohol, taking drugs, watching porn, gambling and so on. The behaviours can compound both the initial and secondary issues around their mental, physical, social and financial wellbeing.

Identity and purpose

Many of these behaviours and resulting life status come to a head in our 40s. This is when the highest average divorce rates occur and, of those suicide rates referenced earlier, it's also highly concerning that 42% of all suicides are men between 40–54.

I believe this is when many men, being outcome-focused, tragically only see one way out; an idea that they have somehow failed at life or are no longer useful; a perception that life hasn't worked out and the best outcome is to end it.

This is of course absolutely not the case and, as famed and highly influential Psychologist Carl Jung stated: 'Life really does begin at 40, until then you are just doing research'. I interpret this as a point in life when we become more reflective and, depending on circumstances, make an assessment of how things have gone so far and what really matters in life.

Typically, younger men seek the superficial outcomes around aesthetics: friend group status, financial success, titles, and overall social status the norm. In my experience within coaching, therapy and supporting men's health groups, around aged 40+, it seems for many to be more about impact, legacy, value to others, and a transcendence of what matters and what will still matter for others and society overall about the life an individual has led.

This results in many wanting to focus on bigger things than themselves: the more impactful, more meaningful parts of life. Therefore, ultimately, I think it is so important that we help all men see there is plenty of time and lots of opportunities for them to have a positive impact, irrespective of how life has gone so far.

Strategies and Awareness

In headline terms, there are many proactive and preventative strategies that can be applied to tackle some of these issues:

- **It's good to talk:** Normalising being able to talk and show vulnerability. Men need different perspectives, so they do not overthink, especially in an overly negative perception of situations.
- **Stronger together:** Creating groups, forums, events and channels for men to widen their perspective. (It is great to see this emerging societally with groups like my very own NXT45).
- **Same old, same old:** Helping men see that by just mixing up social circles (a hobby of some type versus the pub or regular social circle) can have a dramatic impact on their outlook.
- **Positive coping mechanisms:** Walking, talking, exploring nature, cardio fitness, lifting weights, creating, completing tasks, reading, breathwork, journaling, meditation – so many such mechanisms can help replace negative coping and even mitigate the need to engage in the behaviour in the first place.
- **Control:** A primary variable for men to improve their sense of self, ability to work out situations and improve their health, is a sense of agency; that they have tools, options, resources and outcomes that

they can influence that can help lead to a plan for a better outcome.

Identity: Who am I and What is my Purpose in Life?

Joe touches on a complex but vital part of the issue we are seeing across men in this modern world: a lot of men are not seeing themselves in descriptions of conventional (and now labelled toxic) masculinity. They feel like their sense of identity is under attack. That is causing a knock-on effect on their feeling of self-worth and behaviour. This two-pronged level of uncertainty is a dangerous mix.

Terms like identity and purpose sound very philosophical in nature and, to a certain extent, they are. A lot of how we feel about the value we add to the world comes from how we see and think about ourselves, and whether we believe there is a place for us.

Allow me to unpack a little bit what I mean by identity and purpose and why it matters to men.

In the life of every man, there comes a time when the questions Who am I? and, What am I here for? demand answers. These are not just philosophical musings as I mentioned earlier, but rather they form the foundation of a fulfilling and meaningful life. Identity and purpose are essential pillars of a man's wellbeing, shaping his decisions, relationships, and contributions to the world. Without these anchors, men may drift aimlessly, risking feelings of inadequacy, despair, and even self-destruction.

Identity Means What Exactly?

Identity is the sense of who you are, encompassing your values, beliefs, skills, and the roles you play in life. A well-formed identity provides a framework for understanding yourself and interacting with the world. All the way back in 1968, psychologist Erik Erikson described identity formation as one of the key stages of human development, particularly during adolescence. However, for many men, questions of identity extend well beyond those teenage years. In fact, as we get older, and often lonelier, the questioning of who we are will rear its ugly head once again.

But why does it matter?

- **Self-understanding**: A clear sense of identity helps men understand their strengths, weaknesses, and aspirations. It provides clarity on what they stand for and what they will not tolerate. In my capacity as an HR professional I talk to a lot of people about their careers and help them try to build a good level of self-awareness. Quite often we talk about emotional intelligence, which in very simple terms is an awareness of how your own emotions impact you and those around you. If you know what you stand for, know what is right and wrong in your values system, and have a set of principles you live by, then life is much easier, especially when you are tested through times of stress or setbacks.

- **Consistency in action:** Knowing who you are allows you to run a thread between thoughts, feelings, behaviours and actions. This consistency builds confidence and credibility in personal and professional relationships. Of course, we cannot just go around doing whatever we want. For a civil society to work, there needs to be give and take with how we approach things. This is amplified even more with our deep and meaningful relationships. Knowing who we are and being aware of how we react to certain situations, allows us a much better chance of building those relationships and being a functioning and valuable member of society.
- **Bounce back ability:** In a world where life sometimes seems like it is continually slapping us in the face and laughing about it, feeling overwhelmed is a normal state of being. Knowing who you are and what is important to you allows you to build a shield that helps deflect some of those challenges or enables quicker recovery should they get through our emotional defences. At work, I often use simple tools that look at how people like to be motivated and build their relationships. You might have heard the

term psychometrics – a simple piece of software that gives people an idea of the things they do well naturally as well as those areas they need to work on for it to become natural. Sometimes I coach people using psychometrics as a baseline, and the data shows there is something happening in their life to compromise their identity. This could be due to something they are working on; someone they are working with, or something outside of work that is impacting their ability to work or live in a way they want to. My go-to question for such people is: What can you do to do more of the stuff that feels natural to you, and you enjoy doing? It is a wellbeing check-in. Conducting yourself in a way that goes against what you believe in or find natural is exhausting, and it leads people to lose a sense of who they are and why they matter. Often my conversations lead down the road of asking whether the person is in the right job, and sometimes they decide it is not and leave to find a job more closely aligned with their personal values.

All sounds great, right? Sure, but in this increasingly complex and confusing world, men are struggling to find their identity, which can be so powerful in shaping their behaviours.

What is getting in the way?

There are lots of reasons why men are struggling with working out who they are. Just to whet the appetite, here are some of my topline observations:

- **Cultural and societal pressures:** Expectations about masculinity can force men to adopt roles that feel inauthentic. Let us pretend for a second that the view of masculinity has not changed rapidly, and that men will just do what men have always done and be the breadwinner, dominant provider and protector of their family. That level of pressure has brought us to where we are today: high suicide rates, uncontrolled mental health problems and fear of expressing true feelings. In addition, society's stance has since shifted, now telling men to be different. It's easy to see the problem guys might face with working out what they stand for.
- **What is a man, anyway?** The fact that the image of what it means to be a man in the modern day has evolved so quickly, regardless of whether it is for the right reasons or not, has sent a lot of guys into a tailspin. If being a man was tough previously, then at least they knew where they stood. Things like changes in expectations around behaviour, career choices, parenting habits etc., all contribute towards causing identity confusion.
- **I want to be like that guy:** Social media and the portrayal of guys, especially online, is also extremely

unhelpful. Seeing influencers, fitness models, porn actors and celebrities living their perceived best life online leads men to draw unhealthy comparisons, causing men to potentially feel inadequate.

The Power of Purpose

While identity answers the question Who am I?, purpose answers Why am I here? Purpose is the reason for your actions and the driving force behind your goals. It is deeply personal and can range from providing for your family to pursuing a passion or fighting for a cause.

Why does purpose matter?

- **Motivation and drive:** Having a clear purpose provides the energy needed to overcome obstacles and stay committed to long-term goals. If you have your eyes on the prize, or you can articulate why you think you are on this earth, then it enables you to stay focused and keep moving forward, even in the face of setbacks.
- **Mental and physical health:** We already know that men are far more susceptible to things like heart disease and are far less likely to seek help for emotional ailments. Interestingly, research by Hill (2016) shows that having a sense of purpose reduces the risk of depression, anxiety, and even physical

health issues like cardiovascular disease.[17] While it might seem philosophical when taken at face value, there is evidence to suggest mind over matter is a valid state and believing in yourself can have a direct positive impact on your physical and mental wellbeing.

- **It's dull but worthwhile:** If we are not feeling our best then getting out of bed can feel like a struggle sometimes. Layer on top of that the stress of work (or looking for work), family life, and what I would term 'adulting' (getting through your to-do list, running errands, completing chores, etc.), having a lack of reason for doing it can make it seem much easier to just pull the covers back over your head, close your eyes and hope it all goes away. Purpose gives meaning to these daily tasks and makes even mundane activities feel worthwhile.

Men often derive purpose from different sources at various life stages. Life is seldom a straight and simple linear journey, and often your best laid plans go in the bin when different things occur unexpectedly. The truth is that our purpose and identity will fluctuate and bend as we move through our life's milestones.

---

17 Hill, P. L. & Turiano, N. A. (2016). *"Purpose in life as a predictor of mortality across adulthood."* Psychological Science, 25(7), pp. 1482-1486.

The things that matter to you as a child and into your teenage years often become irrelevant once you reach adulthood. Teenage years are often about exploration and self-discovery when we have grand plans to conquer the world or go into space. Once we hit adulthood and things like bills, family, relationships and careers start to become more complicated, our sense of who we are and why we are here starts to change. As men go through later life, reflection begins and, depending on how your life has panned out, feelings like regret could make an appearance. But as older adults, men will likely start caring more about legacy, spending more time on personal interests, or simply just surviving.

The key message here is that no matter the stage, a man's purpose is never static. It evolves with his experiences, priorities, and circumstances. But without an understanding of this and our emotions, it can feel like we lose parts of ourselves as we get older. Of course, the healthy way to think about it is that we evolve with life, and that is normal and perfectly fine.

Feeling purposeless can be devastating. It often manifests as apathy, restlessness, or despair and can lead to harmful consequences and poor decision-making. I will share more examples of my work as a police officer later in this book, but over the years I have been too far too many suicides of men. They are always equal parts sad and shocking but the thing that always gets me emotional is when we are searching for any notes left behind. The reason we look for that information is to try and rule out any foul play but also to try and give the family who has been left behind some semblance of an answer as to why this has happened.

Two of the most common words that I have found in suicide notes from men are 'worthless' and 'hopeless'. Of course, purpose and identity are also important to women, but it seems the profound impact on those men with a lack of identity or purpose is often more devastating.

Questioning your identity and value in life does not mean you are having a mental health crisis or considering suicide. If you are in otherwise good health, have positive relationships, good self-awareness and positive coping strategies, then it is just a natural part of your existence. However, for men, often their concerns are compounded by the sacrificing of friendships, bottling up how they are feeling, ignoring health concerns, and getting involved in negative coping strategies like drinking, gambling or drug taking.

Finding Identity and Purpose

The journey toward identity and purpose is deeply personal, but in my experience, there are some simple things you can put in place to help. These strategies for action come mostly from my experience as a coach in the corporate world, but also my own personal journey with working out who I am and why I am here.

- **Reflect on your values**: Your values are the core principles that guide your life. Ask yourself:

  1. What do I believe in?
  2. What do I stand for?
  3. What would I like others to remember me for?

  Reflecting on these questions can help you define your identity and inform your purpose.

- **Set meaningful goals:** When coaching, I often use the phrase 'If you do not know where you are going, all the roads can lead there'. Purpose often emerges from setting and pursuing meaningful goals. Break these goals into smaller, actionable steps, and celebrate progress along the way.

- **Cultivate relationships:** Relationships can provide both identity and purpose. As a partner, father, son, brother, or friend, your roles in others' lives give you a reason to strive for better. Surround yourself with people who inspire and challenge you. Equally, I have found that surrounding yourself with people who have an opinion that you value is also helpful.

- **Contribute to something greater:** I outlined at the beginning of the book the difficult time I had during 2024. While it was undoubtedly tough, I made the choice to let it inspire me to make a change. Purpose often comes from serving others or contributing to a cause larger than yourself.

- **Seek professional help:** If feelings of purposelessness or identity confusion persist, seeking help from a therapist or counsellor can provide clarity and support. Therapy is not a sign of weakness but rather a tool for growth and self-discovery. This is something GenZ are much more comfortable with than past generations. Personally, I actively see a therapist on a semi-regular basis as it helps me keep things in perspective. We do not need to wait for a crisis to happen before seeking expert support.

Perry Timms, a famed and powerful voice in the HR world who champions positive change in the world of work through his business, shares his story below, outlining how his sense of purpose and identity have been directly impacted by his relationships and family circumstances. The HR community votes for its most influential people each year. These are the people who are actively trying to make a positive difference to the workplace through their thought leadership, networking and passion for doing things better. Alongside being voted HR's Most Influential on several occasions and being part of HR's Most Influential Hall of Fame, behind the scenes Perry's personal life and purpose are defined by the love he has for his wife. Perry shares his own thoughts and tips on retaining your identity, while still having purpose in this complex world.

Perry's Story

We've had homo economicus (profit orientated), homo politicus (power orientated) and even homo digitalis (tech orientated). Now we should also be looking at homo curans (people who are care orientated.

In the animal and human kingdoms, caring for others was mainly done by the female of the species. UK figures for 2024 show only a 5% take-up of Shared Parental Leave (SPL) by eligible men. Despite the ever-growing offer of this policy by employing organisations, 'carer' and 'male' are less prevalent word couplings than 'carer' and 'female'.

Yet 41% of those who care for another adult, likely their life partner, are male. Though women are still the dominant percentage at 59%, this is a significantly higher portion when compared to SPL.

Why is that?

My own experience is exactly that: I've become an adult carer (homo curans). And in a bizarre, potentially random, connection, I'm the second successive male adult carer in my family – my dad having cared for my mum for over 20 of her final years. And of his family, two of his three brothers did/are doing the same.

With my aunts and uncles, severe debilitating conditions hit them in their 50s, 60s and 70s. With my mum, a gradual clustering of rheumatoid arthritis, type 2 diabetes, renal issues, visual impairment and, eventually, what caused her to pass away – heart failure. My dad (and his two brothers) was fortunately capable, either semi or fully retired, and they could turn their time, effort and energy from work into care.

What's different for me from my dad and uncles is that it's happened much sooner in my life, as my wife was diagnosed with multiple sclerosis in 2006 aged 39. For the first three years of living with MS, my wife was able to work full-time and seemed largely unaffected by it. However, seven years later, the gross tiredness and struggles to walk for any reasonable distance without impact were evident. So, part-time became her working pattern. Three years after that, she had to give up working completely. Since then, it's been a mix of increasing domestic chores for me to where we are now: a constant state of care and reliance. MS depletes people, primarily of their energy and then their ability. It's also difficult to manage, as some things are sudden while others gradual.

Caring can be challenging. Knowing what to do and how to be—whether to encourage someone or risk sounding flippant and toxic-positive—makes caring for an adult a trickier proposition than it might be when caring for a child. However, it's still nothing compared to the daily challenges people who need care experience every hour of every day.

What have I learned as a male adult carer in the last five years?

- **Recognise when it moves from additional tasks to actual care:** It sounds obvious, but there's the initial subtle difference and an increasingly obvious shift from helping more to actual care. The reason for this is the need to 'contract' with each other differently, from a list of chores, to knowing what attentive, flowing care needs to be. It's useful and important that you and the person you're caring for name that shift and recognise what it needs from each of you.
- **Listen and explain:** Caring for an adult is more about life's psychological and psychosocial elements than just knowing how to handle mobility and hygiene. It can be difficult for someone being cared for to rely on another person. So, opening up a more expressive form of dialogue builds understanding and confidence in each other.
- **Practice tolerance and patience:** Luckily, I am tolerant and patient, yet I find myself stretched and tested regularly. Carers are not simply there to provide physical support. They are counsellors, coaches and sense-makers. That can sometimes mean you're the outlet for frustrations and anger from the person being cared for. You may pull a little hard on the

sleeve of the jacket you're helping someone get on, and this may imbalance them and they may react a little curtly. It's understandable and all part of the learning process. Equally, you are not an emotional punchbag, so there is a red line.

- **Retain your identity in addition to being a carer:** It can feel like a very consuming shift from partner to carer – more time is needed for the intimate and challenging aspects of life. You can be up for this, proud of being able to help and assimilate it into your life.

It can also be difficult to balance and integrate. I started out with a long-standing ambition: to build my own enterprise. One year after setting that in motion, my wife decided that continuing to work was no longer viable for her. Not exactly how I'd have drafted the risk-averting plan!

However, with the risk comes flexibility and choice. It's probably easier for me to adjust to owning my own business than having a corporate job where I have to answer to their terms. It's important for me that I still enjoy watching live football with my dad and following my interests, like music and other sports. But all this is balanced with being a carer.

In essence, being a carer of another adult is probably not what we'd put on our bucket list of things to aspire to in life. Yet, as we find ourselves living longer lives, it is far more likely that we are going to become adult carers, and life partnerships will literally be in sickness and in health, as the traditional matrimonial pledge goes.

While not a goal we set ourselves, there is enormous fulfilment and worth in caring for someone impacted by life events.

In many cases, it is also a joint responsibility. Working together, learning together and sharing the challenges coherently and collaboratively, shifts life partnerships into different interdependencies and definitions of care.

My ultimate piece of advice when faced with being an adult carer?

Know the story of you.

Who are you? And what core values and principles do you uphold and even admire in yourself?

My story is about deriving joy by being generous to others, plus respecting and honouring duty and obligations. I've learned to lean on and channel those things when becoming a carer and having additional responsibilities. It's another dimension of who I am.

Caring for another adult needs to be an extension of who you are.

Chapter 3:
I am Desperate to Belong

Let me start this chapter with an alarming stat that comes from a workplace research report by employee engagement company Reward Gateway. This specific research, called the *Workplace Connection* report, surveyed thousands of HR people and non-HR employees in 2023 and found that as many as one in four people experience frequent loneliness in the workplace.[18]

25% of us feel lonely frequently. Isn't that shocking and sad?

Having a sense of community and therefore connectivity to like-minded people is so important but easily overlooked. Especially where men are involved. What about making men feel like they also belong?

---

18 Reward Gateway. (2024). *The Workplace Connection Report: How to Build Connected, Emotionally Resilient and Productive Teams*. Available at: https://www.rewardgateway. com/uk/resource/workplace-connection-report [Accessed 18 September 2024].

Isn't a sense of connection and community important to everyone?

What do I mean by community?

I am talking about people with a similar set of experiences, interests, likes and dislikes as you. It's also made up of individuals who have their own unique perspectives on the world that should be celebrated and shared. We all have this natural desire to want to be part of something, to feel like we belong.

In his fascinating book, *Social: Why Our Brains are Wired to Connect*, Matthew D. Lieberman talks about social pain being as real as physical pain.[19] If we get a snub from someone, a cruel word that we don't like, or a rejection of our opinion, it hurts us.

We use phrases like 'he broke my heart' or 'that really hurt my feelings'. Being lonely or feeling like you do not have a place in the world is a feeling that drives people to do things they would not normally do. Does a sense of loneliness become a contributing factor to poor physical and mental health in men? Of course it does.

In chapter two, I talked about how men are far less likely than women to seek help for medical conditions. It's hard enough to encourage guys to open up and seek help even when they have a strong unit or social circle

19 Lieberman, M. (2015). *Social, Why our brains are wired to connect*. Oxford University Press. Oxford

around them. For those alone, it is even harder. The chances of noticing something being different in behaviour or lifestyle is higher in women because women are generally better at having sustained and regular social interactions.

If a man distances himself from others and has no one around to support them, monitor them or talk to them, it can easily become a slippery slope to poor health. Importantly though that feeling of needing to feel you belong does not go away, even if you are living on your own and perhaps feel like society has left you behind.

We can talk about extreme behaviour here to bring this to life.

In an article published in the *Journal of Clinical and Diagnostic Research* in 2014, which explored the relationship between loneliness and psychiatric disorders, they found that lonely people suffer more from depressive symptoms, as they have been reported to be less happy, less satisfied and more pessimistic.[20] The same research shows that loneliness and depression share the same common symptoms such as helplessness

20 Mushtaq, R., Shoib, S., Shah, T. and Mushtaq, S. (2014). *Relationship between Loneliness, Psychiatric Disorders and Physical Health. A Review on the Psychological Aspects of Loneliness*. Journal of Clinical and Diagnostic Research. Available at https://doi.org/10.7860/jcdr/2014/10077.4828. [Accessed 13th November 2024]

and pain. Sometimes people feel like they are so alone that there is no point in them being here or the pain is too much to deal with. So, they decide to end their life, as to them, there is no value to it.

For a lot of people, that feeling of needing to belong drives them to seek connections. This could be anything from social groups like the local book club, sports team or joining a gym. For others, it might be more contentious, seeking a sense of community with people with radical views. This could be anything from the existence of aliens, conspiracy theories or end-of-the-world type groups, all the way to radical extremist terrorist organisations.

In the UK, in 2024, there was a period of real disruption that saw far right extremist groups take to social media and ultimately the streets to 'protest' about immigration in the UK. I use the word 'protest' though the behaviour reported to the general public was more akin to violent disorder and serious racism.

I am sure this was bubbling under the surface for a while and quite often all these extremist groups need is a self-perceived valid reason to light the touch paper and justify their actions. This was sadly brought about by an awful attack in the Southport area in the northwest of England in which a 17-year-old boy attacked a group of children who were attending a Taylor Swift-themed dance party with a knife, killing three children and seriously injuring many more.

Rumours started circulating online that the profile of this attacker was an illegal immigrant, and he was even given a name. This led to an uprising of far-right protests taking to the streets and attacking mosques, immigration lawyers and hotels that housed asylum seekers. This quickly turned violent with hundreds of police officers being injured, businesses being looted and unprovoked attacks on members of communities being commonplace.

We have seen similar patterns of behaviour in the USA, especially during the presidential campaign of 2024 between Trump and Harris. One of the things that Trump led heavily on was the uncontrolled flow of 'illegals' into the USA via the Mexican border. He went a step further to blame a lot of the violence, murder and rape on this particular group of people. One memorable story that got a lot of attention was Trump telling the world that some illegal immigrants from Haiti have been killing and eating family pets in the town of Springfield. Despite being debunked as untrue by the local council in Springfield, the story gained traction. Trump fans and far-right groups used it as a reason to protest and get their voices heard.

Why does it matter about the rumours being circulated online?

Research outlined in Ofcom's annual Media Nations Report in the UK, found that just 48% of young people tuned in to live TV each week in 2023. This represented a drop from 76% in 2018. Those aged between 16–24 were found to watch just 20 minutes of television a day, but when it came to video streaming and sharing platforms, 93% spent on average one hour and 33 minutes watching content.[21] On the whole, young people are getting their information from the internet. They are using platforms like TikTok and YouTube to consume what they believe to be factual information and spreading that disinformation onwards for others to fall into the same trap.

There is a healthy debate raging about children's use of social media, with more adults than ever coming down on the side of the fence that agrees social platforms like TikTok, X and others should be banned for anyone under the age of 16. This is one to keep an eye on as the Australian Government has announced its plans to do exactly that – in 2025, the intention is to block social media access for those under 16.

I think this is an interesting argument and one that has plenty of 'right' answers on both sides. There is no doubt that accessing unfiltered and vast amounts of information online can be dangerous. However, is there a better argument for a different course of action?

---

21 www.ofcom.org.uk. (2023). *Media Nations 2023*. Available at: https://www.ofcom.org.uk/media-use-and-attitudes/media-habits-adults/media-nations-2023/.

Possibly. I remember someone giving me an analogy years ago when there was a huge debate in the UK about knife crime. Sadly, knife crime is on the rise in the UK, with weapons readily available, and more often than not chosen by young people (young men in particular) to 'keep them safe' in whatever gang dispute they are having. Seldom is there a shift I am on in the police where there is not some form of call to someone carrying a knife or someone being threatened/stabbed.

The analogy though is something to ponder. The tool itself, in this case a knife, can be used to seriously injure someone or take their life. That same tool can be used to butter bread for a family or chop up some vegetables for a delicious meal. So, is it the knife that is the problem (the tool) or the intent behind its use (I know there is a very big difference between a bread knife and a zombie knife, but you get my point). If I apply that same logic to a social media ban, is it the tool itself that is the issue or how it's being used or understood by young people?

The swathes of positive educational information online for children and young people makes it difficult to introduce an all-out ban. However, but I can also understand the fear of social media and the negative impact it has on people's lives. A tough debate which I am sure will continue to split opinion for years to come.

Back to the riots in the UK. The rumours about the alleged attacker's identity were called out by police as being 'fake news' with them taking the unusual step of confirming the attacker was born in the UK. But it was too late; the news had spread, the dam had burst, and a process had begun that took a long time to rectify.

The Labour Party promised swift and decisive action and, importantly, consequences for those participating in the violent disorder. This led to the police making hundreds of arrests all over the country for a variety of offences, including posting harmful content on social media which aimed to incite violence.

At the time of writing this book, more than a quarter of people charged in relation to the riots across the UK were aged 21 and under. All males. Maybe that isn't shocking given what we now know about how young people consume their information. Perhaps a little harder to comprehend is the fact that a good proportion of these people were 16 and 17 years old, with the youngest person to be charged just 12.

What has happened to these young men to lead them to resort to such violence?

Going back to the feeling of needing to belong, one mum read out a statement in court as her young son was being sentenced. She said that her boy was a good young man, (helped her out at home as she was disabled), and has not been in trouble with the police before. She could not understand what had made him do this.

Another mum who had two of her sons charged and convicted for an attack on a library in Liverpool in which items were stolen and a large amount of damage was done, thanked the judge for the sentence, as she thought it would be harsher. She even said one of her sons was spurred on by the other as he had asked his sibling for help to cause damage to the library.

A mother of a young man who was sentenced to time in prison for posting hateful comments on social media encouraging people to attack a hotel housing asylum seekers, said that she was shocked by his behaviour and could only guess that he had been 'swept up' in it all.

This is what can result from the need for a connection; the danger of not having proper role models. This is something we need to address for young men and boys. From where are they getting their information? To whom do they look up to? If they have a deep-seated and intrinsic desire to feel like they belong, if society is not offering them suitable options, perhaps rather inevitably they will seek inappropriate connections. There will be plenty of groups counting on the disillusionment of young men, ready to take advantage.

Where are the Role Models?

International Men's Day 2024 had a theme which focused on positive role models. The annual event, which aims to shine a spotlight on specific men's topics and create a space to celebrate the guys in the world, thought it was important to focus on this topic. Maybe it is a sign of the times, the concept of role models seemingly more relevant than ever before.

We are a product of our environment, right?

The raging, never-ending and frankly irritating debate of nature versus nurture has rumbled on forever and will likely continue to do so until everyone reading this book is long gone. Who knows what the answer is. For the sake of a balanced view, let's just say everyone is partially correct and it's probably a mixture of our genetics and external influences.

I am no genetic scientist, so I want to explore the idea of the external influences (nurture) in more detail by discussing the importance of role models in modern-day manliness, and the often-hidden impact of followership.

Let us assume that the rise of social media influencers, fake news, divisive politics and extremist groups are having a negative impact on our young men and boys. Assuming comes with its risks, but given what we know about how information is consumed by young people I think the assumption here is correct. I mention young men, but I am not ruling out the impact that the influencer has on all men. Typically, though, the one thing older guys have on their side is life experience and a maturity to at least distinguish between nonsense and reality.

In chapter two, I talked about people going down the path of least resistance, and in our current landscape, we only have two options for men and boys: option A (be less man and be more woman) and option B (be more man and forget the progressive changes that have been made to reclaim your rightful place in the world). With only these two viable options ever really talked about, it is easy to see how crafty and semi-switched on 'role models' can take advantage of a confused and increasingly marginalised generation of males.

The riots we just discussed were mostly brought about by commentary online. Truth be told, we are living in a world dominated by a few key voices that manage to communicate to so many males. Online influencers use their various platforms to entice fandom and empathy for people looking for a listening ear, and compete with each other to get the most followers, likes and shares. Content has become increasingly more extreme, and we are in an age where it's very difficult to work out what is real and what isn't. Truth often does not matter when there is a good story to be told.

Though I would not refer to these so-called influencers as role models, I am certain a lot of people in the western world would; a digital world that targets us 24/7.

Our politics in the western world is verging on laughable, and you do not need to look too far to see the type of impact it is having. We can see this most vividly in the USA. Trump has won his second term, despite being a convicted felon, using racist rhetoric to stir up fear and rolling back years of gender and sexuality progression.

There is this hypothetical question people have some fun with:

'How would you describe our world to an alien who just landed?'

If I was to talk to an alien who just landed on planet Earth and told them the story of Donald Trump winning his first term in the White House and how that ended, the alien would rightly ask: "But why was he re-elected? Didn't you learn anything from the first time?" My answer would cause that alien to promptly jump back into their spaceship and tell his overlords not to bother taking over our little planet as we are all crazy!

But facts are facts. One of the key things that won Trump his second term as the most powerful man in the world was the high turnout of young male voters who signed their cross next to his name on election day. So, if we thought we could hide from the online influencers and be OK, we were wrong. We literally have policymakers who divide society, criticising each other and trying to win votes by making people feel a certain way about the world they live in. The group most likely to gravitate to this are, yup, you guessed it, men.

It is easy to get sucked into the spiel from the loudest voices or the ones with the power – I understand how and why it happens. They say things that make sense to confused people; they create disinformation that resonates with the disenfranchised, who are not particularly bothered if it's true; they sell merchandise, promise change, and convince people they are the saviours of our broken world.

But here is the thing: those loud voices are representative of a really small minority. Often, it is easy to forget all the other voices that have something useful to contribute.

It is not the celebrities or politicians we should be listening to but the 'regular' men who, for the most part, despair of some of the news stories and scandals that involve other guys. These are the men who will do everything they can to support all parts of society; these are the men who will cross the road at night to avoid a lone female thinking she is being followed. These are the men who are having conversations with their children, brothers, students and friends every single day.

The real role models we should pay attention to are the hard-working fathers, sons, brothers, uncles, friends and co-workers. These are the voices that have the potential to influence our society for the better. They are neither rich nor famous; they are just guys who give a damn about the influence they have to the people in their social circle.

For young men and boys to grow into functioning and productive members of a diverse society, they need positive role models around them from an early age. The challenge is displaying the behaviours and language that make a lasting positive impression on those young men desperately seeking validation for their feelings and thoughts. That is why the International Men's Day 2024 campaign for positive role models was so important.

If you are a man reading this and you have influence over other guys in your life, please stop and think about the man you want him to become. You have more power than you realise, and your actions have consequences.

For any young men reading this who are wondering where their positive role models are, they are all around you. If you are reading this and thinking, I literally have no one in my life that is positive, then just look out to your community. Things like youth clubs, community centres, sports teams, running & boxing clubs and gyms all exist. Ignore the loud corrupting voices and instead choose a path that allows *you* to become a future role model. Behave now like the man you want to become.

How About Men and Communities in the Workplace?

I shared some statistics at the beginning of this chapter from employee engagement company Reward Gateway that showed many employed people feel lonely. Reward Gateway conducted another piece of research on the power of appreciation.[22] This was looking at how important it is for organisations to value those working for them, rather than just seeing them as employees.

The research encourages us to see that appreciation is about seeing someone for who they are, not just what they do – the human being as well as the employee; the good and the not so good.

Sounds really simple, doesn't it? If we treat people as people rather than an anonymous paid employee, they are more likely to work harder for you and your business. In fact, Reward Gateway share a statistic from the Haas Business School in the USA (which specialises in the link between human science and business performance) that states human beings who feel appreciated in the workplace are likely to be 43% more productive than those who do not.

In my role within the HR industry, I know first-hand that finding great people is tricky; retaining them for a

---

22 Reward Gateway. (2024). *The Economic Value Study*. Available at: https://www.rewardgateway.com/uk/resource/economic-value-study [Accessed 18 September 2024].

long time and maintaining their productivity is even trickier. Employees have much more choice now than they ever have before, and people make their employment decisions on a wide range of factors.

Rather than having jobs for life, prospective employees are looking at things like social value (the positive impact an organisation has on the local community), climate impact (the difference a company is making to the planet), and social connection.

A research report called the *Appreciation Index* describes the top five reasons people might feel appreciated in the workplace.[23] The relationship with managers and wanting to be praised by the organisation both appear in the list, but the most interesting one to me is wanting to feel like you belong.

People want to connect to the values of a business, but they also want to feel seen for who they are. They want to know that their voice matters, and their opinions are valid. They also want to know that a business will take care of them and those important to them. Having the confidence in an organisation that allows someone to be their authentic selves, is a sweet spot for organisational culture.

---

23 Reward Gateway. (2025). *The Appreciation Index | Reward Gateway*. Available at: https://www.rewardgateway.com/uk/ resource/the-appreciation-index [Accessed 12th January. 2025].

How does this apply to our concept of community and connection among men?

If we take the typical workplace as an example, through the diversity, equity and inclusion movement over the past few decades, employee resource groups (ERGs) have seen a boom. An ERG is a safe space for people to connect inside organisations and share experiences, life lessons and, ultimately, create awareness for whatever their chosen topic is.

Typically, and rightly so, the majority of these groups focus on areas that historically have not had the voice they deserve in society and/or have been marginalised for various reasons, including race, gender, sexual orientation, and social background.

A lot of businesses have these spaces set up for areas like social mobility, the LGBTQIA+ communities, accessibility, and for better gender equality for women. The term 'ally' is often included in the title to make sure they are inclusive. Such spaces also encourage those who do not identify with one of the groups to still join and take part, or at the very least be educated so they can also be a voice for change and acceptance.

What we do not often see in organisations is an ERG specifically for men. Despite the inclusive purpose behind the ERGs and their powerful symbol for promoting diversity and belonging in the workplace, there is a glaring gap in the schedule for men who will likely be asking, What about me?

That question is by its very nature quite divisive. I understand the possible negative reaction from parts of society when I, a white, middle-class man in the western world, asks, What about me?

There are of course a lot of men out there who form part of the underrepresented community. For this point, I am talking about straight, white, cisgendered men. Should men settle for the privilege of being an ally to the underrepresented groups? Or should men also be included in the inclusion debate? There are various arguments for and against making this more common. Let's look at a few of them and see how they stack up.

Men Should be a Part of the Equality Conversation

Is it possible to further the gender equality debate without men? By engaging men in the conversation around equality, it will not only help to further educate them and build a sense of wanting to be part of the change but also create the deeply ingrained need to be part of it. That will strengthen the idea of allyship and everything that goes with it.

I remember attending an International Women's Day webinar at work that told the stories of some inspirational women within the organisation. After about 45 minutes of listening to the career struggles of some of the women on the panel, their advice to their younger selves, and their hopes and dreams for the future, it was time for an audience Q&A.

The first question was: 'Where are all the men?'

With the exception of a few, including some of the senior leadership team sitting as part of the panel as the overt allies, there were very few men in attendance. Now, on face value you might look at this and think, bloody men, they do not care enough to even attend a session on International Women's Day!

From my point of view, the lack of male attendees was not due to apathy. And it certainly was not due to opposing the event itself. No. The business I work for has one of the most progressive cultures of which I have ever been a part. It puts diversity, equity and equality at the heart of its strategy and is inclusive and thoughtful in everything it does. It has a slightly younger average age of employee than most businesses, averaging around 27.

I think the reason there were so few men that day was simply because they didn't feel it was their place to turn up to an International Women's Day webinar on the career struggles of women in the business. It wasn't malicious or ill-intended; it was likely a lot of, 'Who am I to join in on this conversation? I am a guy. I don't want people to roll their eyes at me.'

This is one of the unintended consequences of excluding males from things like ERGs – they feel awkward, and they believe they are not a credible voice in the conversation around gender equality because the argument, up until now, is that men have spent a lifetime getting ahead of women just because of the sex they were born with.

Us Guys Have Troubles Too

There are just some things that guys would prefer to talk to other guys about. This is not about keeping secrets or plotting to take over the world. It's just easier to talk to other men about men's problems. They can come at it from a place of empathy rather than sympathy.

If we accept, as per the general theme of this book, that men in 2024 are struggling with the concept of what masculinity is and how they relate that to themselves and their own feelings and behaviours, the emergence of safe spaces to chat about all of those things with others who may be thinking something similar, surely can only be a positive thing?

'Not all men want to talk about this stuff, Chris.'

This was some feedback I got when discussing the idea of setting up an ERG just for men. I was not quite sure how to take it, though I had to concede the point. There might well be men out there who don't want to discuss their feelings or learn how to check their testicles for lumps. There are probably some men out there who do not want to talk about their behaviour or the impact that it might have on those around them. I understand.

Safe spaces for men to talk about their feelings are not mandatory–some men might not want to talk–but I am certain there are a lot of men who just don't know how or have never been given the space or confidence to do so.

The lofty ambition is that eventually every man at the very least wants to be educated on men's issues like male cancers, male behaviour, and how to be a better version of themselves. If they choose to take part in the conversation, that would be wonderful. If they choose just to listen and take it away to think about, then that is wonderful as well.

The assumption that not all men want to talk about their feelings is actually part of the problem. Assuming that guys who historically have not said much or expressed their emotions want to stay that way, is dangerous. The suicide rates are a simple yet shocking set of statistics that suggest this way of thinking has not, or is not, working. So, let's rewrite the script and encourage every man to talk.

November each year sees men all over the world attempt to grow a moustache or beard to raise awareness and money for men's health charities and good causes.

This is all about having an external reminder (on your face) that some things are specific to men and ignoring it would just be silly. Typically, Movember raises money for charities that focus on men's mental health, suicide prevention, and male-specific cancers and ailments.

Joe Gaunt, who we met earlier in the book, ran a series of sessions for my business during Movember that focused on men's health topics. He shared statistics, information on testosterone, and his own experience as a psychologist before taking questions from the audience, made up of a pleasing mix of men and women.

Questions from the women included such things as how could they help their fathers or sons with things they were struggling with, and how to start conversations with guys without it feeling like an intervention or making it awkward?

Maybe it is a shift in the narrative around the importance of supporting our guys, but I do not think that even a few years ago, running a session dedicated to men only issues would have happened – it would have been too controversial. But progress is progress.

If you are reading this and you have some form of influence in your organisation on wellbeing, benefits and that type of thing, then just cast your eye around your workforce. What percentage is male versus female? I'd imagine you have a lot of guys working for you, and in some industries it's more likely to be far more male-oriented. In fact, if you are in typically male-dominated industries like construction or trade, then this applies to you even more.

You cannot and should not ignore men's health through fear of causing upset. I am confident that if told correctly, the story of why the men in your business matter just as much as the women will be well received by both genders.

Won't the Men's Groups Just Take Over?

In our quest for gender equality, could men having their own space cause the male voice to dominate the conversation around inclusion, and potentially drown out female voices?

The concern of this happening makes sense. Afterall, for thousands of years the male voice has indeed dominated the conversation, made the decisions for society, created the laws and, ultimately, brought us to the position we are in today.

But this is a very different world to that which existed in previous decades and generations. I think we have come too far in the rise of the women's movement to allow this to happen. I also do not think the vast majority of men would want to dominate the conversation again. The progress that has been made is remarkable in such a short space of time. Guy's will be looking around and seeing their mums, sisters, friends and any other female in their lives having much more independence, confidence, opportunities and freedom to be themselves than in previous decades.

In fact, this current generation of young men and teenage boys will not have known anything else. They only know what they see and hear from those around them, and from their male role models or peers.

So, if that is true, then the risks associated with not giving men a space to connect with other men to talk about male-specific issues and concerns, far outweighs the concern of setting them up.

If the safe spaces do not exist, then the young men of this world won't have anywhere to learn from other than from social media or their elders. The elders who do remember a world of inequality. This becomes a role of the dice, as it then leaves it to chance as to whether guys have the right people in their lives to open up to, learn from and, ultimately, imitate.

Chapter 4:
Domestic Abuse

Away from writing books, podcasts and various other extracurricular activities, I am a volunteer police officer in Brighton on the UK's south coast. Brighton is a vibrant city with a mix of every sub-culture society has to offer, with its two universities, visiting tourists, foreign language students, a big homeless population, and an easily accessible hotspot destination for hen and stag dos. The city also has lots of drug use and mental health concerns to contend with.

For those wondering what a volunteer police officer is, let me explain. In the UK, we are called Special Constables. In very basic terms, we are fully trained, kitted out, and warranted like our regular colleagues, but we do it for free. Committing a minimum of 16 hours a month (probably the equivalent of two shifts) means we stay current in our skillset and can fit it in around other commitments like work and family.

I have been a Special in Brighton for 10 years, working mostly with the response team. This means we respond to 999 calls, anything from murders to lost children, from suicidal people to fights in the pub. And everything else you could possibly think of.

The majority of the incidents I attend are related to one of two things (and often linked). Firstly, mental health concerns. This typically manifests itself as someone acting oddly, feeling suicidal, has locked themselves in somewhere, gone missing, or become violent – all as a result of an underlying mental health condition. The second most common type of call is related to domestic abuse.

Domestic abuse, often referred to as intimate partner violence (IPV), has become a significant public health and social issue across the western world. Over the last few decades, the recognition of domestic abuse has grown, with increased awareness, reporting, and government responses to try to tackle it.

Despite these efforts, the rates of domestic abuse have remained alarmingly high, and are often inflated around significant events like the World Cup or even the Covid-19 pandemic.

But domestic abuse is not just violence. It can and does take many forms, some of which are hidden and difficult to prove from a legal point of view. Away from the violence, domestic abuse can also include sexual abuse, psychological (by way of coercive and controlling behaviour), emotional (cutting people off from family or friends, for example), or financial (controlling how much money someone has access to).

In this chapter, I aim to explore why domestic abuse exists, why it is on the rise, and why statistically men are far more likely to be the abuser rather than the abused. I will share some stories from my time as a Special Constable and also outline the implications of domestic abuse for the perpetrator, victim, families and our local communities, suggesting ways how we, as men, can and must do better to stop the domestic abuse epidemic from getting worse and continuing on to the next generation.

History Leaves a Scar

Historically, domestic abuse was largely hidden, often dismissed as a private matter. In many Western societies, that traditional view of manliness and the male being the stronger gender supported the notion of male dominance in the household, effectively silencing victims, predominantly women, and perpetuating a culture of 'see no evil, hear no evil'. The feminist movements of the 1960s and 1970s were instrumental in bringing domestic abuse to the forefront of public consciousness, advocating for not just legal reforms but the establishment of shelters and support services for victims. These movements also highlighted the need for societal change in attitudes towards gender roles and violence.

However, despite positive advances, much more openness, better reporting, and much more overt support for victims, domestic abuse continues to be a real problem. There is no doubt that the reasons for this are complex and multifaceted, involving socioeconomic factors, cultural norms, and individual behaviours. On top of these, in recent years, the issue has been exacerbated by global crises, including economic recessions, social isolation, and the Covid-19 pandemic, which have all contributed to an increase in domestic abuse incidents.

Locked Down, With Nowhere to Go

One of the most significant recent factors contributing to the rise in domestic abuse is the Covid-19 pandemic. Lockdown measures, intended to curb the spread of the virus, had the unintended consequence of trapping victims with their abusers, while simultaneously cutting off access to support networks and services. This situation created what many experts have termed a 'shadow pandemic'.

Statistics from various countries highlight the severity of this issue:

- In the UK, domestic violence killings doubled in the first three weeks of lockdown in 2020, compared to the average rate in the previous decade. Calls to domestic abuse helplines increased by 25% during the first lockdown.[24]

- In France, reports of domestic violence rose by 30% during the first lockdown in March 2020.[25]
- In the US, data from police departments across several cities indicated a 20% increase in domestic violence reports in the early months of the pandemic.[26]

These figures underscore the devastating impact of the pandemic on victims of domestic violence, as well as the limitations of existing support systems in times of crisis.

While working with the police during the pandemic, a large proportion of what we had to deal with was a mixture of covid rule breakers (think garden parties and sitting on benches), people having a mental health crisis, and domestic abuse.

24 Havard, T. (2021). *Domestic abuse and Covid-19: A year into the pandemic*. House of Commons Library. Available at: https://commonslibrary.parliament.uk/domestic-abuse-and-covid-19-a-year-into-the-pandemic/.

25 OECD. (2020). *Women at the core of the fight against COVID-19 crisis*. OECD Policy Responses to Coronavirus (COVID-19), OECD Publishing. Paris. Available at https://doi.org/10.1787/553a8269-en

26 Peterman, A., et al. (2020). *Pandemics and violence against women and children*. Center for Global Development.

We know that domestic abuse shows itself in many forms, but the one on show the most during lockdown was physical abuse and violence. You do not have to take a massive leap to understand the simple reasons why this was the case. Government laws literally locked perpetrators inside their houses with their victims, and the understanding was that it was illegal to leave the house other than for short periods of exercise.

Obviously, the police actively deal with domestic abuse, and of course it would be silly to think the Covid-19 restrictions had any impact on whether police would attend a call for help. However, in times of confused legal understanding and a fear of getting ill by being outside your bubble, you can understand why some victims might think staying inside was their only choice at the time. In addition to that, being trapped in a home with your abuser makes it extremely difficult to make a call for help.

We also see a spike in domestic violence during big cultural events, specifically football tournaments when England plays, and loses. Of course, not all men are abusers, and not all men react to things like a loss in football by attacking their partner. But the stats are the stats – an unacceptable number of men do.

So, if you are reading this and you are one of them, what are you doing? And if you are reading this and thinking, that's ridiculous, I would never behave that way, monitor your own emotions, and also those of your close mates during these types of events and have a word in their ear if their temperature is rising too much.

Why are Men More Likely to Commit Domestic Abuse?

There is no doubt that men are far more likely to be the perpetrator of domestic abuse rather than women. There are a plethora of reasons why but it is important to also say that men suffer domestic abuse, which perhaps is not reported nearly enough and certainly not talked about, enough.

The following words are from Mark Brooks OBE. Mark is an authority figure on government policy in the UK on topics including male health and domestic violence and he gives us his view on the subject.

Mark Brooks OBE: Men Don't Talk About Domestic Abuse... But Are You Listening?

It is a common question in the overall field of domestic abuse as to why any victim, male or female, does not reach out for support and/or talk. That includes more formal channels such as the police or a GP, or alternatively, a friend, family member, work colleague or neighbour.

In terms of male victims, there are two issues at play: masculinity and society.

On the masculinity issue, there is always the nature versus nature debate – the interaction of how men are programmed at conception and later socialised. Notwithstanding where anyone fits, men internally feel they have a provider/protector role, they need to be/want to be of service, and fear judgement of not being strong, social and respected. When it comes to being a victim of domestic abuse, this plays out in several ways.

Firstly, men cannot comprehend being a victim of domestic abuse, even more so at the hands of a woman. So, when they are, they have this enhanced sense of shame, failure, and embarrassment because it undermines their sense of being a man. They are not in control of their destiny and are not strong. They also think they are the only man in the world that this has ever happened to.

Even more so when, as likely, there are size differences. One man I have worked with was 6ft 4ins and in the armed forces. His wife was 5ft 5ins. His fear was how will that look to the outside world when he declares he is being physically harmed?

In 2022, research from the Domestic Abuse Commissioner really shone a light on how masculinity plays out. It showed 74% of male victims wanted support for the partner who was abusing them (47% of women said the same).[27] In essence, the men were more concerned about the person harming him, than their own safety.

Anonymity at first disclosure or the provision of information is really important, too. This plays out in male help-seeking more widely. Information on websites is crucial, including toolkits, action plans, and also hope. These are featured on the ManKind Initiative website because they tap into masculinity. There is a list of real-life survivors' stories (names and locations changed). They talk through the experiences these men had, how they left, and that they are doing well now. Men need to be told clearly what to do, that other men have gone through it and, importantly, that there is hope.

Three in every five men who call the ManKind Initiative helpline only do so because it is anonymous. The same percentage also state that the helpline is the first time they have told anyone. Many are looking for validation, as they are not sure they are a victim, not sure who to talk to and, importantly, want reassurance about how people will react

---

27 Domestic Abuse Commissioner. (2022). *A Patchwork of Provision How to meet the needs of victims and survivors across England and Wales*. Available at: https://domesticabuse commissioner.uk/wp-content/uploads/2023/02/DAC_Mapping-Abuse-Suvivors_Summary-Report_Feb-2023_Digital.pdf.

Building from that is the societal issue, namely how society thinks.

Society does not expect men to be victims of domestic abuse; it is not part of the narrative around domestic abuse. Therefore, some do not react in the way they should. They do not take the male seriously or he has to work hard to convince them because they cannot comprehend that he could be a victim (for example size difference).

In addition, they can have a lack of intuition or personal curiosity. That is, even though the signs are there, they are not conditioned to think about it so do not see them. For example, their son has a new girlfriend whom he has moved in with five miles away. Over the next year or so, he stops sending birthday cards, stops going to the football or popping round for a cup of tea. Do the parents think he is just 'loved up'? Or do they think he is possibly in an abusive, controlling relationship?

The point here is that on the flipside of masculinity is how society views men and how in, turn, perceived masculinity prevents them speaking out.

This is the nub of the problem. We cannot expect more men to talk if we are not providing them with the space to do so. This includes not being curious enough to think men can be in an abusive relationship and then not supporting them when they do. It is a two-way street. It is one of the reasons I always push back on themes of 'men don't talk' when equally, we need to be listening just as much, if not more.

Traditional Gender Roles

Mark touches on a key point which is a general theme of this book. Giving men the space in which they feel safe enough to open up about how they are feeling, in a non-judgemental and supportive environment is a crucial intervention which does not really require much money and certainly is not massively complex.

The rest of this chapter will be focusing on the reasons why men are more likely to be abusers rather than be abused. Households are much more diverse than ever before, and people have much more freedom to identify in whatever way they want to (there is still lots of work to do in this space). For full transparency, I will be talking from the angle of and sharing examples from typical male and female relationships and family dynamics.

Domestic abuse is a behaviour rooted in power and control, and understanding why men are statistically more likely to commit such acts requires an exploration of several interrelated factors, including biological, psychological, and socio-cultural influences.

From a young age, historically boys and men are often socialised to view aggression and dominance as acceptable or even desirable traits. I am not saying that playing with toy guns and watching wrestling are factors in turning young boys to violence, but it must have an impact on how they see their role in society and the use of aggression, even in a playful way.

While we can acknowledge that it is evolving, traditional gender roles reinforce the idea that men should be the 'head' of the household, exerting control and authority over women and children. This socialisation process can lead to the internalisation of beliefs that justify the use of violence to maintain control, particularly if you have your authority or ego challenged.

We have looked at the idea of 'toxic masculinity' already, and this is often discussed in psychological and sociological research, highlighting how rigid and harmful definitions of masculinity can contribute to violent behaviours. If you happen to be a man who subscribes to the traditionalist and conservative views of yesteryear, then you may well feel not only comfortable, but entitled to assert your self-perceived notion of dominance through aggression, particularly within intimate relationships where power dynamics are more pronounced.

If the only options you have on the table are option A or option B, you can easily see why men might revert to type, especially in situations where they feel the need to assert themselves.

A Guy's Head Can Be a Tricky Place to Be

Do men suffer mentally from things that women don't? I don't think it is as black and white as that, but there are certain psychological conditions and traits that are more commonly associated with men who perpetrate domestic abuse. While not an exhaustive list and certainly not an excuse, these can include:

- **Narcissism:** A personality disorder characterised by a need for admiration and a lack of empathy for others. Narcissistic individuals may resort to violence when they perceive that their authority or self-image is threatened.[28]
- **Antisocial personality disorder (ASPD):** Individuals with ASPD often exhibit a disregard for the rights of others and are prone to impulsive, aggressive behaviours. This disorder is more frequently diagnosed in men, which may partly explain their higher rates of violent offending.

---

28 Cohen, L. J. (2018). *Narcissism and domestic violence.* Psychology Today. Available at: https://www.psychologytoday. com [Accessed 12 December 2024].

- **Anger management issues:** Men are more often socialised to express anger outwardly, sometimes leading to violent outbursts. Not all angry men get violent, but usually this anger is one factor driven by other things which we will look at next. Difficulty managing anger and stress, particularly in the face of relationship conflict, can precipitate acts of domestic violence.

Trying To Stay Numb

In the chapter looking at men's health more broadly, I talked about how studies have shown that men are more likely than women to abuse alcohol and engage in heavy drinking and drug taking, usually as a coping mechanism. Going back to my role in the police, there is absolutely no doubt in my mind that drunk or drugged people act in a way that if they were to watch themselves on TV, they would be embarrassed. Quite a lot of the drunks that I come across, especially in the town centre on a Saturday night, are very friendly, loud and obnoxious. Some still take instruction and go home to sleep it off and regret their decision to have another shot of tequila at 2am.

However, there is also a big proportion of those drunks, usually men, who act in a way that amazes me. They get into verbal arguments over the tiniest things, and when two male egos come together, it often turns into a fight. Add the likes of cocaine to the mix or any other drug that they might be recreationally taking or indeed are dependent on, and people turn into the worst versions of themselves.

That is how they act on the street when there are lots of people watching them, including the police. The mind boggles when thinking about what then might go on behind closed doors.

There is a well-established link between substance abuse and domestic violence. Foran & O'Leary (2008) write in their paper *Alcohol and Intimate Partner Violence* that alcohol and drugs can impair judgement, reduce inhibitions, and escalate aggressive behaviours, which increases the likelihood of domestic violence incidents.[29]

Not Being Able To 'Provide'

Economic hardship, particularly among men who feel societal pressure to be the primary breadwinner, can lead to frustration, anger, and a sense of inadequacy. These feelings can be exacerbated by unemployment and/or the inability to make ends meet. Could this lead

---

29 Foran, H. M. & O'Leary, K. D. (2008). *Alcohol and intimate partner violence*. Clinical Psychology Review, 28(7), pp. 1222-1234.

to some men expressing their frustrations through violence against their partners?

Economic stress is particularly potent in relationships where traditional gender roles are strongly upheld, as the inability to fulfil the expected role of provider can be deeply emasculating i.e. I feel like I am less of a man, so I am going to take it out on the person closest to me.

The economic downturns of the 21st century, including the 2008 financial crisis, the economic impacts of the Covid-19 pandemic, and the economic fallout of the war in Ukraine, have exacerbated these stressors, leading to an increase in violence within the home.

For instance, research from the ONS indicates that areas with higher levels of unemployment and poverty have higher rates of domestic abuse. In the UK for example, data shows that women living in households with an annual income below £10,000 are four times more likely to experience domestic violence compared to those in households earning more than £50,000.[30]

The rise of feminism coincided with the rise of a movement to try to put women on an equal financial

---

30 Office for National Statistics (2018). *Women most at risk of experiencing partner abuse in England and Wales - Office for National Statistics*. Ons.gov.uk. Available at: https://www.ons. gov.uk/peoplepopulationandcommunity/crimeandjustice/ articles/womenmostatriskofexperiencingpartnerabuseinengland andwales/yearsendingmarch2015to2017.

footing as men. The need for companies to comply with things like Gender Pay Gap Reporting is becoming more common, and the gap is thankfully closing. However, in places where economic freedom has yet to rise for women, economic dependency can trap victims in abusive relationships. Many victims, particularly women, may feel unable to leave their abusers due to financial constraints, lack of access to resources, or fear of having nowhere to live. This economic entrapment perpetuates the cycle of violence and makes it difficult for victims to seek help or even talk about it.

Cultural Beliefs

Cultural norms that condone or trivialise violence against women also play a critical role in perpetuating violence against females. In some communities, domestic abuse may be minimised, rationalised, or even accepted, particularly in cultures where male dominance is deeply ingrained.

In addition to what most people would assume we mean when talking about domestic abuse (i.e. a male against female), the rise and awareness of honour-based abuse and violence also needs to be talked about. This is usually when perpetrators perceive that a relative has shamed their family and/or community by breaking their honour code.

Interestingly, in the UK, honour-based violence or abuse is not a specific statutory offence. It instead acts as an umbrella term for various offences including forced marriage, female genital mutilation, male child preference and male privilege.

According to the Metropolitan Police, people who carry out honour-based abuse are often close family members but could also be extended family or even community members.[31]

This cultural backdrop can provide a permissive environment for domestic abuse, as it may discourage victims from reporting abuse and reduce the social stigma against perpetrators. In fact, in some cases, reporting it would bring further shame and likely lead to social exclusion from a community or family.

While on duty one day, a call came through to the control room that a female had reported her partner for locking her out of her house and threatening her if she tried to get back in. Sussex Police have a policy on calls that seem to involve a 'domestic' element that requires attendance as quickly as possible and a sergeant to be made immediately aware to make sure it gets the care and attention it deserves.

---

31 Metropolitan Police (2019). *What is domestic abuse?* | *The Met*. Police.uk. Available at: https://www.met.police.uk/advice/advice-and-information/daa/domestic-abuse/what-is-domestic-abuse/.

I always try to read the basic information on calls beforehand to try to get a sense of what I might be walking into. It is also normal for police officers to check the history on that address or the people living in it in case there are any warning markers for things like violence or any similar calls made in the past. When we did the checks for this particular call, nothing was flagged. This was fairly unusual, as most incidences we attend of this nature have some form of history with the police. Obviously, everyone has to start somewhere, and this is where this particular couple were starting their relationship with the police.

The female who had made the call was at her parents' house, so we went to meet her to try to work out what had happened, and how the police could help.

Being locked out of your house, in which you are both legal tenants, is not a matter for the police – it is what we call a civil dispute. But threats are unacceptable, so we attended to get her version of events. We record everything on body-worn cameras and for this particular job it was a good thing that we did. This lady was from a culture that supports arranged marriages, and one in which the man typically has the control.

We asked her to tell us what happened. After an initial silence, the lady then spent 30 minutes relaying what appeared to be years of control and, ultimately, domestic abuse. She had never spoken about the things she was sharing, but once she got started, her brain raced so fast to remember all these different things that happened it was difficult to make sense of it all, work out a timeline, and keep her on track. Sometimes in the police, you just need to give people the space to talk freely and for them to feel safe to do so.

She told us stories of how she was tracked on her electronic devices (stalking), forbidden from going out with her friends (coercive control), bought lavish gifts in the early days (love bombing) and refused access to her own money (financial abuse). But she had never been physically abused. She emphasised this point several times, as if she was trying to make sense of it all and trick herself into thinking that her partner wasn't an abuser.

When we asked how long it had been going on for, she told us 12 years, the same length of time she had been married.

We asked what had prompted her to call the police now, and what had stopped her from calling the police in the past. Her answer was chilling, but not surprising given the circumstances of the family setup: she was afraid to tell us; she would be shunned by her community and her family; she would be left with nothing if she told us anything. She called us now as she had a son and was worried for his safety. She was willing to accept the community reaction for the sake of her boy.

We can talk about statistics and theories around things like honour-based violence, but this was a real example of how cultures can have an impact on the lives of partners, family members and friends. They would rather suffer to save their reputation than live a free life.

Incidentally, it took nearly the entire 10-hour shift to get her account, get his account and, ultimately, arrest him for stalking and coercive control. The result? No further action taken!

Why? I hear you scream.

Somehow, overnight, she decided she did not want to support any prosecution, and her family were not willing to support her version of events either, despite witnessing some of the behaviour. There was no evidence and no one willing to give us any.

The plus side?

He was now on notice and on our police systems with history against their address, so should something else happen in the future, we now know where it all potentially started.

It Can Happen to Me or Mine

As we progress through the changes in the role of a man in modern society, we cannot forget the multiple generations of traditional gender roles that many young men today grew up with.

I talked about role models in the community chapter. But how does it apply to domestic abuse? Ever heard of the expression 'Do not tell me, show me?'

Men who have experienced or witnessed violence in their own childhoods are more likely to perpetrate domestic violence as adults.

Hines and Saudino (2004) talk about the cycle of abuse. They say that "*it is a well-documented phenomenon, where individuals who were abused or witnessed abuse as children may normalise violent behaviour and replicate it as an adult*".[32]

I would know this as the 'cycle of violence' and it underscores the importance of addressing childhood trauma as a means of shutting down the hamster wheel.

Not everyone who has been abused themselves or been in an environment where it happens, becomes an abuser. Though life is shaped by our environment, it is never a foregone conclusion just because of our circumstances. Life is defined by a series of choices and decisions. These choices often set us on a course in our life, but the choice is still ours. So, accountability is important. It would fall into the category of a 'cop out' or an excuse if people use their upbringing to justify their behaviour in adult life.

---

32 Hines, D. A. & Saudino, K. J. (2004). *Intergenerational transmission of intimate partner violence*. Journal of Family Violence, 19(1), pp. 19-33.

Let me give you a real example from my own life. I have a sister who is three years older than me. We both grew up in Northern Ireland, same parents, same problems with our family, same physical setting and, I believe, the same opportunities. Our lives have taken very different paths. I would class my childhood as complicated, and in fact my therapist described it as 'messy'.

At the age of 16, my sister moved to London to live with Dad's mum (the fact I refer to her as Dad's mum rather than Nan gives you a little insight into the family dynamic) and closed off all communication and relationships with me and my mum.

My parents are complex characters – my dad is an ex-prison officer suffering from PTSD and my mother, a self-confessed alcoholic who doesn't have any interest in changing (it's been that way as long as I can remember. I will talk more about that in the addiction chapter). My sister chose to move away from the family and has firmly played the victim after a series of poor life choices, which have ultimately led to her having a limited life in lots of different ways including socially and emotionally.

My choice was to take all the anxiety, fear, trouble and confused teenage years and use those feelings to power me into my adult life. I chose not to let it determine my outcome but instead to take control of my own destiny and make it on my own. There is no doubt that my upbringing has shaped my perspective on the world, made me guarded with relationships, and caused me to feel a certain way about friendships, but it has not defined who I am as a person.

What Has Policy Done to Try to Stop Domestic Abuse?

Over the past few decades, successive governments have implemented a range of policies and legal frameworks to address domestic abuse. These include protective orders, specialised domestic violence courts, and funding for shelters and support services. Additionally, public awareness campaigns have been launched to educate the public about the signs of domestic abuse and encourage victims to seek help.

As I am writing, police forces across the UK are trialling dedicated domestic abuse call handlers in the contact centres. These are people who are specially trained, with advance knowledge of domestic abuse aimed at helping callers immediately with sign posting, advice and also to rate the risk for other services outside of the police.

Police have additional powers: more detailed forms to complete to test the risk of the abuse escalating, and regular input on changing the understanding of abuse through dedicated training.

A really great example of an awareness campaign is the White Ribbon campaign in the UK. Starting around mid-November, it aims to educate and raise awareness on the impact that men and boys have on women and girls through their behaviour and actions. It's designed to shock as well as create empathy, sharing real stories so women feel they have a platform to talk about something often hidden, and that men can see the impact of abuse.

Of course, a lot of guys when exposed to such campaigns declare they would never abuse a woman so don't need to be educated about it. That is true, most men would not behave in a way that would cause women or girls to fear for their safety. But all men should *care* that the statistics show the majority of domestic abuse is perpetrated by men. Perhaps many of the abusers themselves once believed they'd never hurt a woman either.

However, despite the various efforts to tackle the problem, there are still significant gaps in the response to domestic abuse. In many cases, the legal system is slow to act, and the burden of proof remains high, making it difficult for victims to obtain justice. Moreover, funding for support services is often inadequate, leading to long waiting lists for shelters and counselling services.

For example, in the UK, a 2021 report by Women's Aid found that one in five women seeking refuge were turned away due to lack of space.[33]

So, if the government or lawmakers cannot make a real difference, what is the solution?

I do not claim to have a magic wand that can fix this, but here are some suggested and practical thoughts to consider when it comes to domestic abuse. Like most things, prevention is much better than cure. How can we stop it happening in the first place?

The Path Forward

The first thing to note is that it will take a lot of different parts of our society coming together, in conjunction with the law, to properly address this. That means using statistics that show men are far more likely to be perpetrators than victims. Men in our communities need to examine themselves and their behaviour. Key areas for action include:

1. **Improved access to resources:** Ensuring that all victims have access to the necessary resources, including shelters, legal assistance, and counselling,

---

33 Women's Aid. (2021). *The Domestic Abuse Report 2021.* Available at: https://www.womensaid.org.uk [Accessed 30th November 2024].

regardless of their background or gender. Anyone who has been a victim of domestic abuse deserves dedicated and timely support to process and rebuild.

2. **Economic empowerment:** Providing financial support and employment opportunities for victims of domestic abuse to help them achieve independence and escape abusive relationships.

3. **Education and awareness:** Continuing to challenge and change harmful cultural norms and stereotypes that perpetuate abuse. This includes comprehensive education programmes in schools and communities that promote healthy relationships and gender equality. This is the prevention – we have to stop it happening rather than trying to fix it when it does.

4. **Stronger legal protections**: Strengthening legal frameworks to ensure that perpetrators of domestic abuse are held accountable, and that victims receive the protection and support they need. There needs to be stronger sentencing to act as a deterrent. The victim and the police can only do so much; the courts need to do their part too.

5. **Research and data collection**: Improving the collection and analysis of data on domestic abuse to better understand its prevalence, causes, and impacts, and to inform policy and practice. It's already complex, but the world is complex and only getting worse.

I know this is all much easier said than done, but nothing changes if we just do the same things. Men have the biggest role to play in all of this. Calling people out on poor behaviour, championing respect for women more broadly, and being aware of how your own behaviour might impact your closest relationships, are just a few things to consider.

Domestic abuse takes many forms. It is possible you may not even realise you are an abuser or are being abused. Educate yourself on typical signs and traits of domestic abuse so you can identify it or seek help. The move towards using the word 'survivor' rather than 'victim' is something also worth highlighting. No one should have to survive any close relationship. Women are fighting back using their voice, but listen guys, women should not have to fight at all.

Chapter 5:
The Image of a Man

We always want what other people have, right?

This is true of a lot of things including our appearance. Looking at other human beings and wishing our abs looked like theirs, our hair was as thick as theirs, our muscles were as big as theirs – all pretty common thoughts and feelings.

But what about when we take that a step further and it is not just about looking at other people and wishing you have what they have? What if it is looking at yourself and disliking what you have? That is a dangerous combination we will explore in this chapter, specifically through the lens of how we look at ourselves as men.

Body image has traditionally been framed as a concern primarily affecting women. However, this perspective ignores a growing and significant issue facing men: the struggle with body image and related disorders. Society's historical view of masculinity, as discussed throughout this book, often emphasises strength, muscularity, and leanness, placing immense pressure on men to conform to the perfect image of a man. The consequences of this pressure are profound, often leading to mental health issues, including body dysmorphic disorder (BDD), eating disorders, and a palpable sense of inadequacy.

Over the past few decades, representations of the male body in the media, and more specifically social media, have become increasingly unattainable. From the chiselled physiques of Hollywood action stars to the hyper-muscular figures in fitness magazines, the portrayal of male bodies has shifted towards an extreme and unhelpful narrative. This media landscape cultivates a toxic environment where men feel pressured to achieve these physiques, often at the expense of their mental and physical health.

Studies have shown that men who are frequently exposed to these idealised images, are more likely to develop negative body image and engage in unhealthy behaviours. For example, a study published in the *Journal of Health Psychology* found that men who regularly consumed media that emphasised muscularity, were more likely to experience body dissatisfaction and engage in behaviours like extreme dieting or over-exercising.[34]

---

34 Agliata, D. and Tantleff-Dunn, S. (2004). *The Impact of Media Exposure on Males' Body Image*. ResearchGate. Available at: https://www.researchgate.net/publication/247839476_The_Impact_of_Media_Exposure_on_Males.

Ever heard of the saying 'Instagram versus reality'?

Put simply, we see videos or images online and take them to be true. But the truth is likely something very different. If a guy posts a picture of himself in the gym changing room, we look at it and see popping abs, big veiny arms and the assumption that this person is a boss who is super confident in their body. We then create a little story in our head about him getting all the girls or boys, he must have a highly paid job, and he probably has no concerns in the world.

That's the Instagram part, the version of that post we consume.

The reality part? They have just been working out, so they have the superficial 'pump' of just using their muscles. They have sought out the perfect lighting in the gym, and it's likely they have taken about 20 pictures and then filtered them to find the one that makes them look tanned and flawless.

For anyone reading this who posts those types of pictures, I am not coming for you. I think if you are proud of your body and are working hard to sculpt it in a way that makes you feel great, then more power to you. It takes discipline, consistency and a lot of hours lifting metal in front of a mirror.

My point here is this: in my experience, a lot of guys who post those pictures online are insecure about their looks. They are seeking some form of validation and are likely frustrated with their own lack of progress. Add in the guy who is looking at it and thinking, *I wish I had that body. It is never going to happen. I hate how I look*, and what you get is a false portrayal seen through a fake lens. It's not real. Plus, such pictures hide real feelings and emotions. This in simple terms creates a narrative from the man seeking what the other has that he is not good enough but what he is chasing is a type of perfection that is actually unattainable.

The Mirror Does Not Lie

Body Dysmorphic Disorder (BDD) is a mental health condition where an individual becomes obsessively preoccupied with perceived flaws in their appearance, which are often unnoticeable to others. While BDD affects both genders, research indicates that approximately 25% to 40% of those affected are men.[35]

Men with BDD may focus on various aspects of their appearance, such as facial features, skin, or hair. However, one of the most prevalent forms among men is muscle dysmorphia, often referred to as 'bigorexia'. This is characterised by an obsession with being

---

35 Cunningham, M. L., Nagata, J. M., & Murray, S. B. (2021). *Muscularity-oriented disordered eating in boys and men.* Eating disorders in boys and men (pp. 21–35). Springer Nature Switzerland AG. https://doi.org/10.1007/978-3-030-67127-3_3

insufficiently muscular, despite often being highly muscular or even overly so. Those suffering from muscle dysmorphia may engage in excessive weightlifting, restrictive diets, and the use of anabolic steroids in an attempt to achieve what they perceive as the 'ideal' male body.

Speaking from personal experience, I have gone through waves of liking what I look at in the mirror and really disliking what I look like. For a time in my mid-twenties, I used to go to the gym five times a week, eat nonstop, and exercise all the time through sports to get myself into a place with which physically I was satisfied. Sometimes I would catch a glimpse of myself in the right light and think, *Yeah, you got this, Chris, all this work is paying off.*

Then I would jump on the scales to validate my muscle gain, and my weight would be the same. The lighting was different in the bathroom mirror, so all of a sudden, that glimpse where I thought I was making progress was an illusion and I was back to feeling frustrated.

That was my inner feelings. Outwardly, this was against the backdrop of my friends telling me that I looked good, asking if I was working out and telling me I was the biggest I had ever been. But it was never enough.

Is this really an issue?

Understanding the prevalence and impact of male body image issues requires examining the data. Recent statistics paint a concerning picture:

- **Prevalence of body dissatisfaction**: According to a survey conducted by the Mental Health Foundation, 28% of men in the UK reported feeling anxious about their body image. This figure rises significantly among younger men, with 48% of those aged 18–24 reporting dissatisfaction with their appearance. Honestly, I am surprised this is not higher.[36]
- **Muscle dysmorphia**: Research published in the *International Journal of Eating Disorders* indicates that muscle dysmorphia affects approximately 2.2% of the male population, with the condition being particularly prevalent among bodybuilders and athletes.[37]
- **Use of performance-enhancing drugs**: A study by the UK Anti-Doping Agency (UKAD) revealed that 56% of those using anabolic steroids and

---

36 Mental Health Foundation. (2019). *Body Image Statistics in the UK*. Available at: https://www.mentalhealth.org.uk [Accessed 18th September 2024]

37 International Journal of Eating Disorders. (2021). *Muscle Dysmorphia in Men: Prevalence and Psychological Correlates*. Available at: https://www.journals.sagepub.com [Accessed 17th September 2024].

other performance-enhancing drugs were motivated by body image concerns rather than athletic performance.[38]

- **Impact on mental health**: The link between body image and mental health is well-documented. Men who experience body dissatisfaction are significantly more likely to suffer from depression, anxiety, and suicidal thoughts. In the UK, suicide remains the leading cause of death for men under 45, with body image concerns increasingly recognised as a contributing factor.

Statistics are cold data. To bring the reality to life, let me explain a story about a couple of friends, both good-looking men, and from a physical appearance perspective, you would think (and I often did), *I wish I looked like them*.

One is 6ft 4ins, and every time we went on a night out, he would get all the attention from the girls. It was really quite irritating (although I was always secretly grateful as I would be terrified if any girls chatted to me).

Anyway, one day this friend made a random comment about being signed off from work for a few

---

38 UK Anti-Doping Agency (UKAD). (2023). *Performance-Enhancing Drug Use in the UK*. Available at: https://www.ukad.org.uk [Accessed 12th December 2024].

months and how great he thought it was. I remember it well as we were playing five-a-side football on a cold winter night, and he just said it in front of our other mates and laughed it off. The rest of my mates laughed as well and thought it was great.

A few months off work, what's not to like?

It bothered me, though. So, when I got home, I messaged him and asked to meet. I had an inkling something was not quite right. We met, and he told me he was signed off work with depression and was not doing so well. (It is interesting how guys interact in group settings versus one-to-ones. I think mob and lad culture sometimes gets in the way and banter replaces empathy.)

After doing a little digging, my friend told me that he really struggled with his appearance. I was bemused that a good-looking man could feel like this. But what other people saw and what he saw when looking in the mirror were two very different things. He hated his appearance. He had no self-confidence or belief in himself. He thought he was super skinny; he felt ugly.

Now to another friend I mentioned. He is shorter, 5ft 7ins, but muscular. He spent lots of time in the gym and always had a tan. On the face of it, he appeared super confident with his body. But for him, maintaining the look was a complete way of life. He ate a ridiculous amount of food, was always conscious about calories, and would exercise continuously (at work he would find scaffolding and do pull ups on the street). He was extremely active and rarely sat still.

Although I never had a proper conversation with him about what was going on under the surface, I suspect something was amiss with his relationship with his appearance. It was addictive, and he would crave working his muscles or running around.

There are worse things to be addicted to than exercise, but it's an underestimated and misunderstood area of addiction which is just as dangerous as any other type of addiction. This is just within my own circle of friends. No doubt, there are many more guys who, in varying ways, struggle with their appearance while presenting a confident front.

Too Many Calories or Not Enough

While eating disorders have long been considered a female issue, a growing body of evidence suggests that they are also a significant problem for men. The pressure to achieve a particular physique can lead to disorders such as anorexia, bulimia, and binge eating disorder. The stereotype that eating disorders are 'women's illnesses' often prevents men from seeking help, leading to underdiagnosis and treatment.

A study published in *JAMA Paediatrics* found that approximately 10% of individuals with eating disorders are male,[39] though this figure is likely an underestimation due to the stigma surrounding the issue. Men with eating disorders often present with different symptoms than women, focusing more on achieving muscle mass rather than thinness. This difference can further complicate diagnosis and treatment, as traditional eating disorder criteria may not fully capture the experiences of men.

Regular gym-goers will be familiar with the terms 'bulking' and 'cutting'. In plain English, it's spending a set period of time eating more calories than normal to build up muscle mass (bulking) and then going through a set period of time being hyper aware of the amounts of calories they are eating, so they can lose fat and become leaner (cutting). This combination means building muscle fairly quickly and then getting rid of the fat that hides the muscle, the outcome normally being someone who has clearly defined muscles on their body.

This is a well-known and well used method for getting the body you want. But just from the simple explanation, you can understand why someone who was suffering with an eating disorder might use a technique like this to the extreme, and possibly to the

---

39 JAMA Pediatrics. (2020). *Eating Disorders in Males: A Growing Concern*. Available at: https://jamanetwork.com [Accessed 17th September 2024.]

point of becoming dangerous for their health, all in the name of getting a chiselled physique.

How Do We Change Our Thinking?

The stigma surrounding male body image issues and mental health remains a significant barrier to treatment. Many men feel ashamed to admit that they struggle with these issues, fearing that it will make them appear weak or unmasculine. This stigma is perpetuated by issues we face in society that equate masculinity with emotional stoicism and physical strength – we have almost become our Roman ancestors again!

However, breaking the silence around these issues is crucial for fostering a healthier environment where men feel comfortable seeking help. Campaigns such as the UK-based CALM (Campaign Against Living Miserably) have made strides in addressing these issues, providing resources and support for men struggling with body image and mental health.

Education in this area is seriously lacking.

The female menopause is a natural change in the hormones and function of a woman's reproductive system, typically occurring in midlife. A lesser-known phenomenon is something called andropause. Sometimes referred to as the male menopause, it is the slow decline of the male hormone testosterone, which impacts every guy. Andropause can happen for some men as early as their mid-30s. In fact, typically from the age of 34, testosterone levels in men start to decline, and this leads to a whole range of potential issues and changes.

Common signs of andropause are things like increased tiredness, lower sex drive, irritation, mood swings, erectile dysfunction, and weight gain. It would not be unreasonable for men in their 30s to experience some of these things but just put it down to something else. Life is tiring, men are under pressure, and they are likely prone to mood swings; guys as they get older do have lower sex drives and possible difficulties getting an erection. But there might well be an underlying medical cause i.e. a drop in testosterone acting as a catalyst to these things, and it could be treatable through medical intervention.

Ever heard the term 'dad bod'? Often mocked in society and between guys, male friends take great pleasure in having some banter about weight and have no compunction telling their mates they have gained some 'timber'. They say it in a way they would never say to a woman. Why is that OK?

I was on a weekend football holiday with a group of my friends in early 2024. Some of us had not seen each other in a while, and most of us had become dads in the past few years and life had been stressful. One of my friends had put on some weight since we saw him last.

Perhaps it was pack mentality, but someone commented, in a 'banter' type of way, and everyone piled on, commenting and joking at every opportunity about this guy's weight gain.

That is not really my thing, and I called them out on their behaviour and told them they were being unkind and were verging on bullying.

'Nah, don't be silly, Chris, it's just us having a laugh,' came the reply.

Lo and behold, while we were waiting in reception to go out one day, we received a group message from this friend to say he was upset with all the comments that had been made about his weight, and he was going to stay in his room for a while to be on his own. He finished the message by agreeing that he had put on weight, as if trying to justify the behaviour of my mates. I told them to apologise, which they did, and all was fine for the rest of the holiday.

In a situation like that, I highly recommend to guys that if you would not say it to a woman, then do not say it to a man. If you are coming at it from an angle of care and concern, then approach it sensitively; do not become a pack of bullies and make your mates feel insecure. You never know what is going on in their head, and your offhand comments could well be the last straw.

To address the growing crisis of male body image issues, society must challenge the narrow definitions of masculinity that have been ingrained in our culture.

Men should be encouraged to embrace a broader range of body types and recognise that their worth is not tied to their physical appearance. Education, open conversations, and support systems are essential in combating the stigma and helping men lead healthier, more fulfilling lives.

It is also vital to remember that every man's experience is unique. I have shared various examples in this chapter of different experiences of body image concerns, but there will be others reading this who do not relate or experience it in a slightly different way. The key here is to foster a culture of acceptance and understanding. We can create a world where men feel empowered to see themselves as being enough and seek help if required. We need to redefine what it means to be masculine in the 21st century.

Next up is a story from Joe. He is a father, a husband and a regular gym goer who, has by his own admission, had a complex relationship with his appearance. The words are entirely his own.

Joe's Story

The Oxford English Dictionary defines body image as a person's subjective picture or mental image of their own body, and how they perceive their physical appearance in relation to how they 'think' it should look.

Body image in today's society is an important pillar in managing one's mental health. While in today's world we are going in the right direction regarding body positivity, there are always still underlying expectations of how we are meant to look. These narratives are driven by social media, reality TV and the mainstream media. I am grateful in a way that social media and shows such as *Love Island* weren't around when I was young, otherwise my body dysmorphia would've been much worse than it already was. Nowadays, it's everywhere, there are literally shows in the UK where you chose to go on a date with someone based on looking at their naked body, and nothing else. If that doesn't scream a red flag with a large sprinkling of vanity and shallowness, then I don't know what does. People are led to believe that those who have a perfect waist, huge biceps, or an hourglass figure are successful and happy, but in my experience, this is far from the truth.

My journey with my body image developed as a teenager. I was an extremely skinny kid. I was sporty to begin with but once I reached 12 years old, I started playing computer games, and it literally took over my life. On a school day, as a rough estimate, I played computer games five hours a day, and even longer at the weekend. I would hardly stop to eat. This continued for about four years until I reached the age of 16. While as mentioned above we didn't have the pressure of social media to tarnish my body image, as a young boy you always have figures you look up to, whether that be superheroes, actors, or sporting idols.

At 16, when I had a good look at myself, I realised I had to do something about my body image (my attention turned to the fact that I was getting zero attention from the opposite sex unlike some of the other guys in my year). I don't know what led me down the path of thinking it must be because I'm skinny that no girl is talking to me but let me tell you this: in my experience, girls care as little about how much you bench as they do about your rune crafting level on a computer game. That amount is zero, my friends.

Eventually my obsession with how I looked started to take over my life. I would say no to family events because I wanted to go to the gym; I would refuse to go out with friends because it would mean drinking alcohol, being hungover and missing a workout. In truth, I lost a lot of friends because of the unhealthy obsession I had with my body image. Anything that didn't align with my goal of creating the perfect body had to go. I really do feel like I largely wasted my youth because of the number of opportunities I turned down – those things that wouldn't serve my purpose of having a good body image. It felt like being in a prison of my own thoughts. There could be no spontaneity in life because I needed to know exactly how many calories I was eating and at what time; I needed to know what time I would train in the gym, and anything else that happened in the day would need to come second to that. I became severely addicted to multiple sleeping pills because I wanted to get as much sleep as possible in order to be able to train well the next day and maintain my body image. I thought if I slept badly, my body would crumble. Because I would wake up every day from what was effectively a self-induced coma, I would lace myself with an extremely unhealthy amount of caffeine so I could perform in the gym. It was a vicious cycle of taking uppers and downers every day. So much so that I ended up having to go to hospital with heart palpitations and jitters.

It was all-consuming and felt like being on a hamster wheel chasing the endless pursuit of perfection and finally being comfortable with my body image. I would wake up, weigh myself, look in the mirror, and sigh. Whether I looked good in someone else's eyes didn't matter to me anymore, I always wanted to look better. It was like any other addiction, be it gambling, drink or drugs – I always wanted more, and I was never satisfied. When I think back, I really don't know what I was chasing, perhaps some validation from peers who were now few and far between? Was it female attention? Was it recognition for the improvements I'd made to my body? Perhaps. Maybe I just wanted to finally feel like I was good at something.

Truth is, no one else cares about it. It's all in your own head; it's a facade. My body image was simply making me feel unhappy and worthless, but if I didn't have that, I had nothing (or so I thought). My entire self-worth was intertwined *with my body image, and I didn't like myself for a long time because of it.*

Years later, the body dysmorphia was still very much there, and I would often ask myself, *Why am I still doing this?* I was then, and still am, in a loving relationship, my partner loves me for who I am, not the size of my biceps, but the deep-rooted link between my entire self-worth and my body image was still very real. It sounds sad to say, but at certain points in my life my body image issues were so bad that I felt like going to the gym and training was all I had. I simply could not fail at this as I had with many other aspects of my life, and due to that, relationships and career prospects fell by the wayside to make room for this obsession. It seemed like it was the only thing I could control, and many other parts of my life were just meaningless in relation to how I looked, because that was literally all I cared about.

After quite a few years of growth and maturing, my body dysmorphia thankfully isn't as bad as it was. I think a big turning point for me, and what completely changed my 'why', was becoming a father.

When my wife and I first found out we were having a baby, my negative body image thoughts were still rife. Although I was first and foremost of course overjoyed, thoughts began to run through my head: *When will I be able to train? How am I going to cook all my food and eat healthily?* (Spoiler alert, I didn't, I probably ate lasagna three–four times a week for the first month of being a dad!) *and how am I going to keep training when I've had such little sleep?* It gave me incredible anxiety at the thought of the looming 'dad bod', which I assumed was a given for any father and felt like impending doom. But the truth of it is, becoming a dad was the best thing that could have happened for me and my body dysmorphia. My perspective completely changed from how I looked, to how my body felt and what was objectively healthy. This change meant I could focus on being a fit, active, and present father, and set a good example for my son, both by being physically fit but also by displaying healthy eating habits.

My perspective has shifted from finding time to go to the gym to spending time with my son and maintaining an active lifestyle around his schedule. If that means going to the gym at 5am before he wakes up, then I'll do it. Furthermore, my son won't remember or care about the size of my chest, but I hope he will remember the time I spent playing and teaching him how to be a man, time spent much better than obsessing over training, eating and sleeping. It has made me a much happier person overall and has really helped me understand that while I do believe one's health is of paramount importance, looking a certain way to impress essentially nobody makes no sense at all.

The final thing I will say on this, is that body image among men is such a serious issue that in 2023 it was estimated that nearly half a million men in the UK aged between 16–50 were using anabolic steroids. This is an extremely alarming amount, the highest the UK has ever seen. Young men especially have such a distorted image of what a man should look like because of things like social media. Men are willing to put their health on the line in pursuit of what they think is perfection because society has made it seem like the norm to have a six pack or a chiselled chest.

My plea to male readers would be to think hard and find your 'why', because if I could go back to a younger self and really ask myself that, I would've realised that so much of what I thought about the link between my body image and my happiness was completely wrong. I think I would've been much happier than I turned out to be in my early to mid-twenties if I had realised that sooner. Having an aesthetically pleasing body doesn't make you better or more of a man than anybody else, and your self-worth should come from a much more loving place than from how you perceive yourself to look when compared to others.

If you asked me to describe my relationship with my body image now, I would say I train and eat well to be fit and healthy for my son, but I definitely won't say no to an almond croissant!

Chapter 6:
Secret Life of Dads

A wife, two kids, a white picket fence – you don't have to go back too far in time to see the version of 'idealism' society ingrained in a lot of men growing up during the '60s, programmes and TV adverts depicting family life as 'perfect'; mums and dad's creating wholesome moments with their children; mum staying at home while dad is out working. Everyone is full of energy, all of the time.

Things started to change in the '80s and '90s on TV with the boom of sitcoms that started to showcase different family dynamics. From *The Fresh Prince of Bel Air*, which showed the chaos created when a young man enters a well-to-do family home in the suburbs of Los Angeles after being sent away by his mum from the mean streets of West Philadelphia, to hilariously chaotic yet often charming *Only Fools and Horses,* which follows the trials and tribulations of Del Boy, Rodney and Grandad making their way in life as an all-male household in working class South London.

One thing that binds such portrayals of fatherhood is the perception that the man is the provider and protector of the family. Seldom did you see the dad showing emotion or weakness and, in fact, the only time you caught a glimmer of vulnerability was when the dad was struggling to earn enough money to pay the bills or keep his children safe.

We know that the typical role of the male in our world has shifted in the past few generations – how does that transition manifest itself in the role of a father? And how have the pressures of being a modern dad likely added to the identity crisis conundrum we are facing today?

I am going to approach this from my own experiences as a first-time dad. This may not be the same for every father but based on my own experiences and those of other men who have shared theirs with me, there is a darker side to fatherhood, especially in the days leading up to the birth and the early years.

A lot of men want and long to be a dad, so I think it's only fair that we get the full picture of what it's really like. Only then can we create a space and provide support during the ups and downs.

The Pressure of Getting Pregnant

From ovulation tests and pre-pregnancy vitamins, to conversations around timing the 'optimum' time for a baby to be born, planning a pregnancy can feel a little clinical and sometimes military in its nature. The pressure of getting pregnant is intense enough without notifications from apps and other new-age technology telling you the optimum time to conceive.

The thing that gets missed in the fury of trying to arrange the perfect time to mate, is the impact the stress of it all can have on a guy. I am talking about the ability to perform on cue and whether your mind and body are in sync with each other.

The conversation around erectile dysfunction (ED) makes most men shudder with fear. While the honest and accurate thing to say is that it's more common than you think, the feeling of embarrassment, usually followed by some form of shame, makes it an issue a lot of guys would rather not discuss.

A 2024 poll by Click2 Pharmacy asked a thousand UK men about their experiences of ED. Nearly 59% of men said they have experienced it at some point in their lives, with over a quarter of them saying it happens regularly.[40] Perhaps a little surprisingly is the age group most impacted, 25–34, the age many men are trying for a baby.

The fear, perhaps being driven by guys, is of not being able to perform when it matters. The truth is men should not feel embarrassed or ashamed if they are

40 Click2Pharmacy. (2024). *Erectile Dysfunction Statistics*. Available at: https://click2pharmacy.co.uk/erectile-dysfunction-statistics/ [Accessed 30th August 2024].

unable to get and maintain an erection. There is plenty of help available and it doesn't actually matter. Erectile dysfunction does happen and is more common than men may think.

But when you have a biological clock ticking and a partner expecting you to play your part in the process, it is a very lonely place to be for any man when ED occurs. In this situation, ED is not just impacting the man but it's having a direct impact on their partner. This only serves to amplify our feeling of shame and embarrassment as well as adding to the guilt. The result makes a man feel less 'manly' and can lead to him overthinking the problem.

Matthew Sloan published an article in 2020 in *Harvard Men's Health Watch* in which he talks about strategies to help overcome the feeling of shame and worry. Number one on the list is to discuss it with your partner.[41]This is a commonsense place to start, and we know communication is a key part to building strong foundations with any partner. If you start hiding things, you get found out or people become resentful.

But where do you start with a conversation like this when you are drowning in negative self-doubt? The first

41 Harvard Health Blog. (2020). *7 Strategies for Partnering Up with ED*. Available at: https://www.health.harvard.edu/blog/7-strategies-for-partnering-up-with-ed-2020111921385 [Accessed 30th August 2024]

place is addressing the issue and acknowledge what has happened. Ignoring it, making a joke of it, or getting angry about it won't solve the problem.

I think the partner plays a key role here because their response will likely decide how the rest of the conversation goes. So, for any partners reading this, listen to what your man is saying, give him the space to say it, and keep encouraging him to talk by being sympathetic and supportive.

And guys, remember this is a common problem, but there might be some underlying issue that needs addressing. Things like excessive drinking, heavy smoking, poor diet and high stress can all have an impact. Taking care of your mental and physical health isn't just good for longevity, it's also good for your sex life and relationships.

TV advertising about ED and products like Viagra (other brands are available) have brought the issues into the open and while it is great that we are putting these types of solutions out there as a quick fix, there is a way to go to make such adverts suitable for the 25–34 age group.

The adverts typically feature seniors and discuss things being delivered in 'discreet packaging'. This is only fanning the flames of the notion ED is a taboo topic for younger men to discuss and perpetuates the myth it only affects the older man.

It might be stress related; you might just be overthinking it; you might be able to resolve the problem simply by talking to your partner. If these factors are not the root cause, however, I would recommend seeing your GP if you are worried. (I know lots of men struggle to get a GP appointment more than they struggle to get an erection, but it's worth persevering and talking about your concerns with a medical professional.)

When your partner tells you it's the optimum time to conceive, you do not need to be a robot and switch on. Even though it might feel a little clinical and forced, try to keep it as normal and loving as it always has been. Relax into it and try to have a good time.

If for some reason, you cannot talk it through with your partner and/or you cannot get that GP appointment, remember that statistically one of your mates, your dad, or your grandad have all probably gone through the same thing at some point. Be that voice of change in your male relationship group and normalise the conversation. No one knows the feelings involved with ED better than other guys who have experienced the same. There is no shame in admitting the problem; you should not be embarrassed. You are not experiencing this on your own.

As an aside, another pressure that comes our way as young men are the unhelpful conversations that people have about having kids. Typically, such pressure comes from people in your friendship group or family circle, people who make the assumption that A, you can have kids, B, you want kids and C, it is their business. It is no one's business but yours. For men wanting to become fathers, these 'well meaning' questions add extra pressure to perform, assessing our progress in a way most of us could do without.

The Lead Up to the Birth

I am not aware of many people who enjoy going to the hospital. Most people are there because things are not going well for them or someone they care about.

Of course, there are exceptions to this general rule and one of those is people attending pregnancy scans they are expecting. For pregnancies progressing as expected/low risk pregnancies, the typical milestones for scans are at 12 weeks and 20 weeks, with midwife appointments scattered throughout to check everything is on track.

The 12-week scan is the first time most parents-to-be see their developing baby and is the first crucial milestone in the gestation process. If you reach this stage and everything is progressing as it should, then the chance of anything going wrong drops significantly. Miscarriage awareness charity, Tommy's, cites that 80%

of miscarriages take place before this time.[42] Undoubtedly, the lead up to this point invokes an uncomfortable feeling of fear and worry; it really is a 'hold your breath' moment as you wait to be called for your turn.

So, what is the role of the guy in this situation?

For me, it was about staying strong, no matter the outcome. This is a general theme across fatherhood – I must stay strong for my partner. You think you cannot show any emotion as *she* needs you. It is physically happening to her, after all.

This is an outdated view of the role of a man and indeed a father that has no place in modern society. But the unfortunate truth is that this is what a lot of dads feel and think, regardless of the toll it takes on their mental and/or physical wellbeing.

For thousands of years, the role of a dad has been firmly set by society. Back in the day, it was to go out and hunt for food to feed the family. Then it became more about earning money to pay the bills. Either way, his role centred around a simple purpose: to provide for his family.

---

42 Tommy's. (2024). *Miscarriage Statistics*. Available at: https://www.tommys.org/baby-loss-support/miscarriage-information-and-support/miscarriage-statistics [Accessed 31st July 2024].

Thankfully, thanks to the Women's Movement and the creation of more equal rights and roles in society over the past few decades, the view of parenthood has not escaped modernisation and evolution. We are much more progressive than we have ever been before, and it's been long overdue. My wife, like plenty of other women, has a successful career, earns a good wage, has purpose in what she does, and isn't financially dependent on me. I am proud of her because of it.

Historically, it might have been tricky to separate the role of a father and a husband; I argue they used to be one and the same thing. Look after your family, whether that be your wife or your kids, be the breadwinner, the provider and the protector.

Now that we have advanced to the point that more women are financially and emotionally independent of men than they have been in the history of civilisation, the role of a father and a husband are still having an identity crisis of their own.

With it ingrained in my psyche from watching my dad, his dad and other male role models in my life growing up, it is no surprise that as I stood in the scan room trying to work out what the images on the screens where, convincing myself that something was wrong (despite having no understanding of what I was looking at), I talked myself into this stereotypical 'be a man' mindset.

Talking to my wife afterwards, with the wonderful and often clear benefit of hindsight, I explained that I was being strong and wanted to be the rock I thought she needed. Turns out that though she appreciated my attempt to look after her, what she would have preferred was for me to be open about my feelings, so she knew that I was feeling the same as her.

I can see how in an effort to not show signs of weakness, a man can inadvertently appear emotionless rather than someone who is struggling to hold it all together. What was I hoping to gain from trying to be stoical? Perhaps a feeling of self-control? Maybe the feeling of 'being a man'? To my wife however, I was shut off, guarded, giving the impression that I didn't care. This is a great example of how the perception of manliness has evolved over the past generation. Women don't need a man to be the strong one. In my wife's case, she was looking for her husband to share her feelings and let her know we were in it together.

There is nothing that prepares you for becoming a dad.

In the UK, antenatal classes provide expectant parents with help and advice in the lead-up to childbirth. As well as NHS provision, a charity called the National Childbirth Trust (NCT) also offer a series of antenatal classes. Smalls groups of pregnant women and/or their partners attend a series of classes with those at a similar stage of pregnancy. The purpose is to educate, offer support and increase confidence during pregnancy, birth and the early stages of a baby's life.

Reviewing this as a first-time father, I can categorically say these classes were heavily weighted towards expectant mothers. With a particular focus on the lead-up to the birth and the birth itself, the NCT tutor highlighted various scenarios that could happen. This included the choice of delivery methods and pain control, all supplemented by techniques to stay calm in the thick of it.

Alongside that is a short section on what to do once the baby arrives (a very short section that does not even scratch the surface!). As a dad, this was the bit in which I was most interested. There is very little I can do with the physical growth of the baby other than support the mum, but once the baby is here, I can play my part.

It turns out, the hour-long session on how to hold a newborn, change a nappy, bath it safely and get it dressed, is not nearly long enough. Once that baby arrives, expect to have a complete mind blank on what you should be doing!

As a clarifier, NCT do run additional new parent classes once the baby arrives, so I encourage you to make the most of that or similar classes if you are able. I only wish more time was spent before the baby arrives getting us prepared.

The Birth

Throughout this book I include real-life stories from different men who were keen to share their personal experiences and journeys. I thought it would only be right if I did the same. So, what follows are my memories and experiences of becoming a first-time dad to my baby daughter.

It is important to say that this was my personal experience of birth. This does not mean that anyone else reading this will think, feel and experience the same thing. However, I am willing to confidently guess that there are a lot of dads out there who have experienced something similar but have been afraid, awkward or ashamed to say it out loud for fear of being questioned about their feelings. Being a man during the birth is a really lonely experience.

I'm led to believe that women have some form of natural ability to forget the physical pain of the birth. This is why they are able to experience it again. Men? Not so much.

I remember every detail about the lead up to the birth, the aftermath and everything in between. It's impossible to forget. Before the main event, the weeks and days before the birth were really eye-opening.

Enter the sweep!

I remember going to the midwife appointments as we got closer to the due date and the midwife offering my wife a sweep. I had heard of this before from other friends but really had no idea what it involved.

In short, the midwife got her fingers and has a good rummage around inside my wife, trying to create friction in the cervix to kickstart the body into labour.

My wife had a few of these and, during the last one, a load of blood and gloop came out; so much so that the midwife called the maternity ward and said we needed to go right away. The bleeding stopped and the midwife was a little less concerned and instead predicted it would be no more than 48 hours before my wife gave birth. We were sent home and waited. This was on a Thursday afternoon. The following night, we were sitting at home, my wife bouncing on her birthing ball, flicking between watching a murder documentary and *Father Ted,* when the contractions started.

This was it. Reasonable panic ensued. My wife was hunched over on the bedroom floor while I tried to count the length of the contractions and how many were in a 10-minute period. The pain was starting to become too much for her, so I called the triage at the maternity ward and was greeted with suspicion:

"Do you really need to come in?"

"Are you sure they are coming thick and fast?"

"OK, well you can come in, if you want, and we will have a look."

I know that for the midwives, childbirth is an everyday event, but this was massive to us – they made it sound a little like we were being an inconvenience.

This wasn't the last time that would happen.

We made it to the hospital around 9pm and went to the delivery suite. 4cm dilated indicates a woman is in active labour; my wife was at 2cm. The contractions were coming quickly, with barely any breaks in between. I asked if my wife could have something for the pain. They gave her some paracetamol and told us we may as well go home and come back as it was unlikely she would be giving birth in the next 24 hours.

Go home? My first thought was, *are you mad?*

They said we couldn't wait in the delivery suite, and if we didn't want to go home, we would have to go to the labour ward and wait. At around midnight, we did just that. They checked her again and she was still 2cm.

I asked them to give my wife some pain relief and told them that the contractions weren't stopping. They gave her a sleeping pill and advised her to sleep, telling her they will re-examine her in the morning. For the next hour, my wife was crumpled on the floor in pain, the paracetamol having no effect. The sleeping pills made her a little drowsy, but they did nothing for the pain. I had had enough, and I went to find the midwife and said something wasn't right. The contractions were literally not stopping.

"Please help us!!"

"It's just like this, darling. Nothing we can do at this stage. It's going to be a long wait so you may as well get comfortable."

I asked if we could at least get my wife into a bath, knowing it is supposed to make pregnant women feel relaxed. After the drama of getting her in and very quickly out, all with no let-up in the pain, I took her to the toilet. It's fair to say at this point my wife turned into some kind of farm animal. From the toilet floor, she shouted that she felt like she needed to push and proceeded to moo quite loudly.

I was totally helpless. No one was listening to me, and I had no idea what to do.

A midwife who happened to be on her break in the neighbouring room knocked on the door and asked if my wife said she needed to push. She confirmed she did. The midwife assisted my wife back onto the bed and checked her cervix. Confirming she was now 6cm, the midwife went to fetch a colleague.

Why had they not been listening to us? Why had she not been offered stronger pain relief after passing the 4cm mark?

Off to the delivery suite we went. By the time we went 200 yards around the corner, she checked again and had dilated to 8cm.

Jesus Christ!

Gas and air were now a permanent fixture in my wife's mouth, but because she had dilated so quickly, with no one checking along the way, all other pain relief was off the table. It was basically too late.

I was thinking to myself, *I really hope this hypnobirthing breathing routine has the same medicinal power as an injection into the spine.*

It does not.

The one thing that the books, NCT classes, podcasts and conversations do not tell you, is how difficult it is for a father to stand by and watch the person he loves most in the world go through this trauma and not be able to do anything about it.

I was so anxious and terrified by what was happening, but really cognisant of the fact that I could not let my wife see how I was feeling. She needed me to be strong now more than ever. So, what did I do? I stood next to her, counting her breaths to try to keep her calm. I held her hand to comfort her and told her how amazing she was.

The truth? I wish I had been anywhere other than in that space at that moment in time. Not because what I was saying to my wife was not true—it was very true; she was a superstar—but I was so scared by what I was seeing and wanted to run a mile.

But I stayed. I kept up at the head end for two reasons: one, my wife had me in a headlock, so I didn't really have a choice and two, I was already worried enough, without seeing the actual physical birth take place. There was nothing magical about watching the birth. This was a horror scene, and I wanted to stay well clear.

From my head-locked position, I did the same as I had done all those months ago at the scans: I assumed I knew what I was looking for and that everything was going wrong. Hearing the midwives whisper to each other, weighing the blood loss on some scales, calling in their colleagues to check something, was extremely frightening.

My head was all over the place and I just thought the worst. The baby was in trouble, or my wife was in danger. Or both.

Eventually, a doctor came in and said that my wife had been pushing for too long without enough progress and had lost a lot of blood. She said they might have to make an incision to make some room and use a suction cup to get the baby out.

The doctor asked my wife if she would consent.

We had already talked about me being the voice for her when she was unable to speak. In fact, we were told very clearly in our NCT class that this is exactly what the man's role was: take charge, ask questions and be the mouthpiece. At this point, my wife's response was, "Get this baby out of me!"

I told the doctor to do what they had to do. The doctor told me it wasn't my body – my wife needed to consent. If I wasn't in a head lock, I would have chucked a bloody pillow at this medic. I understand that Doctors are trained to remain calm in high pressure situations. I would rather a calm doctor than one who is flapping. But bed side manner is a thing, and I couldn't help but ask myself; why are these people so cold? Can they not see the distress everyone is in?

My wife mumbled her agreement and on we went. But this time a neonatal nurse entered the room with a special unit to take the baby away in the event of an emergency. If my head wasn't spinning before, it was now.

Though this is normal procedure for assisted deliveries and falls into the category of 'just in the case', it wasn't explained to me why they were there, so I just presumed the worst. I was so angry with how this whole thing was being played out. I was terrified for my wife, and I was aching to sit down after standing bent over for four hours.

At 5.33am, my daughter finally arrived. I saw she had lots of hair. I heard her crying and just stood there, in complete silence; not moving, not feeling.

I was in total shock. She was here; she was alive. She was my daughter. But just like when I first heard the heartbeat, I didn't feel how I thought I should. I barely looked at her.

What the hell is wrong with me? was the overwhelming thought I had in that moment. Instead of being flooded with happy hormones, I was numb and distinctly lacking emotion. I can confidently say, now several years have passed and I can reflect on the experience with a degree of detachment, that how I felt was perfectly OK. There was nothing wrong with me, and what I had just been through can make people react in all sorts of different ways.

Just like a lot of the other personal stories shared in this book, I am going to offer my own top tips for each part of the fatherhood journey.

For the lead up to the birth, here is what I would highlight:

- **It is not a comparable experience:** Often men and women have this debate about the most painful thing: childbirth versus being hit in the testicles with a ball. Watching my wife going through the trauma of birth was deeply unpleasant and I cannot imagine the pain. However, my experience as a husband was painful in a different way. They cannot be compared to each other, any more than the physical pain we experience. Men and women experience childbirth in a way unique to them. Both should be respected.
- **Be strong but be realistic:** I can say now that my determination to be strong for my wife was absolutely the right thing to do. But I wish I had talked about my feelings much sooner after the birth to help me process what I had been through as well.

- **Women might forget, but men don't:** There is no shame in admitting how difficult this whole thing is for fathers. The trauma of seeing what you see and hearing what you hear sticks with you. It is 100 per cent OK to not be OK with it.

I Am Responsible for A Real-Life Baby!

The story goes on…

As I stood there not really being able to comprehend what I was seeing, I was snapped into reality when the midwife placed Orla on my wife to see if she would feed right away. My wife was exhausted, was still losing blood and the doctor was trying to stitch her up. She asked me to take Orla and sit on the chair with her so she could rest for a while.

How do you even hold such a newborn baby?

The midwife passed her to me, and I just did the best I could. That pretty much sums up fatherhood. As I sat with Orla on my chest, I was just trying to take it all in while also hoping she wouldn't cry as I had no idea what I was supposed to do. After about 10 minutes, the midwife asked me if I had clothes, nappies, a hat, etc., for her.

Of course, we had been preparing for this moment for months. We had bags full of every sized vest and babygrow, copious amounts of snacks for my wife and I, blankets, formula. *What a stupid question!* I thought.

"Where is it?"

Oh. I had left it all in the car, in the car park, which was about a 10-minute walk away. Upon coming into the hospital, I thought I would have lots of time to go grab the bags. No rush. I got that wrong.

I broke the news to my wife that we didn't have any of her stuff and I had to go to the car to grab it. Orla was put into the little basket, and I started the walk through the hospital back towards the car park.

This was about 6am on a cold September morning and I had been awake for almost 24 hours. As I saw other expectant parents making their way into the hospital (with their bags), I couldn't help but feel a little smug that our labour was done. I also felt sympathy for the men as I knew what they were about to experience.

When I got back, the midwife asked me if I could feed the baby as my wife was trying to rest. She may as well have asked me to do a triple somersault in the pike position while humming a song in Chinese. I literally had no idea how to feed Orla, how much to give her, how to hold her, or how to wind her afterwards.

So, I asked her to do it so I could watch. She begrudgingly agreed. I watched intently – she made it look so easy. She manoeuvred Orla with ease and surprising robustness. (Much more firmly that I was expecting. I was terrified of dropping her or making her cry.)

The next step was trying to dress Orla. Trying to place tiny arms and legs into a babygrow when you have never done it before is like mental gymnastics, taxing a brain already in overdrive.

But I did it; I didn't really have a choice. This is another key lesson from fatherhood: no matter how difficult everything seems, you don't really have an option but to get on with it.

As the day progressed, various nurses and doctors returned to check on Orla and my wife, conducting lots of different tests to make sure everything was all right. I swear every time someone new came to run a different test, my heart stopped, hoping it was not bad news. I guess that perceived lack of feeling I had had for Orla started to subside. I really cared; I really hoped everything would work out.

My wife had lost so much blood that they were not sure if she needed a transfusion. We waited all day for the test results and eventually they confirmed no transfusion was needed but she had to stay in hospital overnight.

I could not stay with her. Covid-19 was still problematical and visiting hours were strict. At 8pm, everyone had to leave. My wife was really upset, struggling with pain, anxious about having Orla overnight, but again there was nothing I could do. I had to leave.

I felt terrible when they told me to go; I felt helpless that I couldn't do more to support my wife. I also felt a massive sense of relief that I could go home to my normal life, to my bed, one last time. As I left the hospital that night, having now been awake for 36 hours, I somehow drove home in a daze and managed to have the last good night's sleep for the next seven months.

You Mean, We Can Literally Walk Out with The Tiny Human?

Waking up in an empty bed knowing my wife and new baby were still in hospital left me feeling guilty. I was really grateful for a peaceful night's sleep, but I knew that the night in hospital would have been scary, lonely and overwhelming for my wife. As well as only recently given birth, losing a lot of blood and not being very mobile, she now had to look after her newborn baby while trying to rest. (I definitely got the good end of that bargain.) As I rushed back to the ward, I couldn't help but wonder what this whole thing was really going to be like. The hard part was done; surely what we just experienced could not be topped.

Erm...

It was time to take Orla home. We took a picture of me carrying her out of the hospital and then the slowest walk in history, to the car, began. Being a new dad meant I had no idea how robust babies are. In my head, she was as brittle as glass; I was treating her so carefully. Turns out babies are hardier than I'd ever imagined.

Upon getting home, we had visitors right away. My wife's sisters and parents came to the house to properly meet Orla and help us out. To say I was grateful is an understatement. They all had kids so knew what they were doing. They kindly offered to hold Orla, make us some tea, change her nappy and make us food. They even helped to milk some colostrum from my wife's breasts using a tiny syringe.

Everyone was really kind and, to be honest, I had no idea how much I needed that support until they all left. Sitting in our lounge as Orla slept was like being in a silent movie. Our first few days were essentially sitting in silence, just waiting for Orla to do something.

I didn't want to breathe too loudly, and I didn't want to move around. We couldn't watch TV. Babies are much easier when they are asleep. When they cry and you have no idea what is going on, it's really quite distressing.

My paternity leave was only for a couple of weeks and my wife was in serious discomfort from the birth, which would last for weeks after. I knew my role: I had to be dad and husband. Chris could take a back seat for a while.

On the aspect of paternity leave, I only had a week, taking a second week as annual leave. I know there are a lot of organisations that offer much more paternity leave, and shared parental leave is becoming more popular. But if you are responsible for parental leave in your company and you are reading this, a week or two is not enough time. To juggle fatherhood and being a husband before then quickly going back to work, is unreasonable. Dads deserve more in terms of options or time to support their partner and get to know their new baby.

Effectively trying to juggle two jobs (employed work and that of being a dad) is a part of fatherhood not often understood or talked about. In the majority of cases, the mother takes maternity leave and is away from work for up to a year, swapping paid employment for full-time motherhood. One full time job swapped for another one. But for men, they go back to their paid job on top of picking up the other full-time job of fatherhood. On top of that, they may have to adopt a caring role for the mother if she is still recovering from the birth. The juggling act is stressful for lots of dads and one I found particularly difficult.

I tried to do everything I could to make it easier for my wife. I really fought hard to keep all my emotions in check; nothing was too much trouble. After all, physically, I was fine. My wife wasn't so lucky.

The first few nights were OK, Orla slept pretty well without too much drama. In fact, she lured us into a false sense of security. She slept on my side of the bed in the next-to-me crib due to the layout of our bedroom. I offered to swap sides with my wife, but she was physically unable to pick Orla up in the early weeks as she continued her recovery from birth. So, when Orla awoke, my job was to pick her up, pass her to my wife and then lay perfectly still for as long as it took to get Orla back to sleep. Babies have no concept of day and night in the early weeks. That is really irritating. We would sit in bed till all sorts of stupid hours just hoping she stayed asleep.

I remember a specific night in the first few weeks which was the toughest night of my life (more so than the birth). Orla wouldn't stop crying, and my wife was exhausted and in so much pain. I was exhausted and didn't know what to do. I had been rocking her in my arms for what felt like an eternity. My shoulders felt like they were on fire and my legs like jelly. Orla wouldn't let me sit down without crying, so I had to keep moving around the bedroom. I was doing my utmost to soothe Orla so my wife could sleep but she wouldn't stop crying.

After an hour of walking up and down the bedroom, we settled her back at my wife's breast as nothing else would soothe her. I felt like I had failed. I walked into our *en suite* and just stood looking in the mirror. As tears rolled down my face, I distinctly remember thinking I hadn't known how tough this was going to be. I just did not feel like I was prepared to be a dad. I wanted it to stop.

I had always wanted to be a father, but the number of irrational thoughts that ran through my head in the early hours of the morning when I was exhausted, were scary. But I have learned that they pass; things do get easier. Even when in that moment in time it feels like the ride is never going to end, you get through the hard nights and try again tomorrow.

After a few minutes, I had no choice but to go back into the bedroom. My wife asked me if I was OK. I told her I was.

I was lying.

But I knew I had no choice than to just get on with it; get through that night and then tackle tomorrow when it came.

For me, there was nothing pleasant or enjoyable about the first weeks as a dad and I am aware that I sound quite brutal. But as my wife always says to me, facts are facts. Survival mode had kicked in, and it would be that way for a while.

This phase of fatherhood was arguably the most testing from a resilience perspective, trying to keep it altogether. The emotions alone are tough and adding on top the juggling act of employment and your new home life is tricky. I'd recommend the following things:

- **Accept the support when it is offered:** There is nothing helpful about pride in situations like this. Lots of people will want to offer support; accept all the help you can get in the early weeks when you're still trying to figure out what you're doing.
- **Babies are gonna, baby:** There is very little point in taking it personally when your baby cries and you can't soothe them. I was not doing anything wrong. Don't blame yourself for babies just doing what they do.
- **Get through each day and night, one at a time:** While at the time it feels like it is never going to end, you just need to get through each day and night as it comes. I actually started planning my days around just getting to the next nap. It makes it much more manageable when there does not seem to be a way out.

Progression and Regression

The words and feelings that came when writing about fatherhood are an honest account of my experience. Honestly, getting that off my chest was equal parts cathartic and shocking. I feel better for it, and it allows me to compartmentalise that period of fatherhood.

As I think back to what came next, my memories and emotions run equally as high.

Everyone always makes jokes about sleep deprivation with babies; I lost count of the number of parents who said it to me when we were pregnant. I always just brushed it off and thought, *How difficult can it be*?

Turns out, tough.

The first few months of Orla being home wasn't too bad. She woke up a few times in the night for feeds, but also went long stretches in between that allowed us to get some much-needed rest.

On Christmas Eve 2022 she slept for eight hours through the night in what I could only describe as a Christmas miracle. I genuinely thought, this is doable now; the hard part is done. What a good sleeper she is.

Erm…

Something changed on 1 January 2023, and it would last for the next four months: the dreaded regressions. I had no idea what sleep regression was or really why it happens but have since educated myself. It occurs during a baby's development as they learn new skills and make 'leaps'. Disrupted sleep patterns also occur for the obvious reasons too, like teething and illness. In simple terms, it could literally be anything that causes a baby to not sleep the way you'd like them to.

Upon reflection, we made a rod for our own back as Orla was exclusively breast fed, only napped when held, and wouldn't sleep unless breast fed first. Knowing we were probably making it difficult for ourselves but also feeling guilty if we were to change what she liked, was difficult. She was just a baby; if she gained comfort from her parents cuddling her and feeling close to us (especially my wife), then that is what she should get.

Throughout January and February 2023, we had to introduce the shift system during the night; we would take it in turns for two hours at a time. That was the window where one of us was responsible for the baby while the other could rest. If Orla was crying so much that nothing would settle her other than being fed, then sadly for my wife her shifts kept going.

When I was able to settle her, the system was essentially walking up and down for ages until we were sure she was in a deep sleep, then try ever so gently to put her in her crib. Invariably she would wake up crying and we would start the process again.

Painful.

We read about sleep training: teaching the baby to sleep on their own. How difficult could it be? Turns out, nearly impossible for us. We paid for a sleep consultant to give us guidance and a schedule. They told us what we should do, the times to do things, the method to follow.

This for the most part just sent Orla into meltdown, and it was too difficult for us to leave her crying. It hurt the soul standing outside the door listening to her crave her parents.

We abandoned sleep training and decided we just had to ride it out. It couldn't go on forever and we just had to dig deep and accept our fate.

Surely it would get better. Fortunately, it did.

From about seven months old, Orla started sleeping much better at night. Looking back, I think the turning point was her ability to roll over and sleep on her side or front. She suffered from reflux so lying flat on her back probably wasn't that comfortable.

I guess to progress, babies need to regress. But those regressions feel sometimes never-ending and relentlessly brutal. These are my key takeaways from that period of my fatherhood journey:

- **This too shall pass:** When you are in the thick of things, it feels never-ending. But as each day passes, knowing that it will get better and this is only temporary, is important.
- **There is no malice from the baby:** Orla didn't know any better. She didn't keep us awake because she thought it was funny. She was uncomfortable, or in pain, or ill, or teething, or going through a leap. She just wanted cuddles from the people she loves the most.

- **Stick with it, it's worth the love:** As she gets older, my love for her has not only developed but has become everything to me.

I could keep going with the trials and tribulations of fatherhood forever. The truth is, as children get older, the problems still exist, just different ones. And crucially, something in you is different too. You either learn to deal with it slightly better or you worry a little less once you know how robust children are.

The role of a father is something that has changed over time and continues to change as society evolves.

Quite a lot of the themes in this book about men's health, addiction, negative coping and stress all have something in common: they are all magnified when they intersect with each other. Typically, one thing seems to lead to the other until they are all intertwined, making it difficult to unpick. The specific role of a father is less set in stone when you take into account the changing nature of the role of a man more broadly, but the stresses and strains associated with being responsible for a little person, with little to no training, should not be ignored.

Of course, there are lots of different types of family set ups – single parents, same-sex parents, adoptive parents, blended families, broken homes, and everything in between. I can only speak from my own experience as a husband with a loving wife, starting out their family journey together. Based on those lived experiences, it is clear to me that the support networks for fathers need to be more visible, and more education is needed for men to better understand how to care for a newborn baby. Fundamentally, society needs to show more empathy towards the struggles first-time dads experience without judgement.

Like a lot of my messages throughout the book, my take on parenthood from the man's perspective does not diminish the effort, pain and trauma mothers experience. Rather, it is about making sure dads can operate at their very best or at least know that how they feel is natural and that support is available should they need it, without feeling ashamed to admit they are not fine.

Chapter 7:
Do Real Men Cry?

Let's start by asking a question about the title of the chapter: are you a real man if you cry?

As discussed at various points throughout the book, having a generalised narrative around what a man is and is not, is unhelpful. The debate around the behaviours, attitudes and actions of a man, although I am sure well intended, add an extra layer of complexity in what is already a complex area.

This chapter underscores the importance of addressing male grief as a distinct and significant experience. It is so important that we continue to challenge societal norms that stifle emotional expression in men, allowing them to grieve openly and heal in ways that promote mental, emotional, and physical wellbeing. The numbers and research make it clear: men need spaces to feel, share, and process grief, just like women.

I echo what I said right at the beginning of the book: we don't need catch-all phrases or sets of behaviour to define what being a man is; it just makes men confused or frustrated if they do not act or feel the way society has defined they should.

The main topic of this chapter is grief. But regardless of what comes next, if you are a guy and want to cry, go for it! If you are a guy and don't want to cry, that is cool as well.

So, what am I talking about when I say grief?

Grief is a universal experience. Experiencing loss, whether that be someone you love or care about, or a slightly lesser explored area of grief (sadness for a previous life which I will explore in more detail later), generally impacts most of us in a similar way. The typical feelings of sadness, anger, frustration, loneliness and resentment are often interchangeable.

Despite the commonality of internal feelings, the way grief manifests itself externally can vary significantly, especially between men and women. As we know, in many cultures men are conditioned to suppress their emotions, often reinforcing a pattern where they suffer in silence. The impact of grief on men, therefore, is often overlooked and misunderstood, as societal expectations dictate that men should be stoic, composed and, above all, strong in the face of loss.

The Unique Experience of Male Grief

Men are often taught, both overtly and subtly, to minimise emotional vulnerability from a young age. Phrases like 'man up' (which is where I got the name for my podcast Hu-Man Up) or 'boys don't cry' can discourage emotional expression and set up an internal barrier to processing grief. When men experience loss, whether it's the death of a loved one, a major life change, or even a deep personal failure, their grief can take on a unique form, often hidden behind a façade of resilience.

Research indicates that men tend to grieve differently from women, not because they feel the loss any less but because of the ways they've been socialised to express or, more often, suppress their emotions. According to a study, *Gender differences in bereavement outcomes and coping*, published in the *American Journal of Men's Health* (2021), men often cope with grief by engaging in tasks or activities, emphasising distraction rather than emotional confrontation. The research highlighted that while women might seek social support more frequently during times of loss, men are more likely to isolate themselves, turning inward to avoid being perceived as weak.[43]

So, even in the mid 2020's, following years' worth of campaigns, research, celebrity openness and a shift in what it means to be a modern man, the research still

---

43 Stroebe, M., Stroebe, W., & Schut, H. (2021). *Gender differences in bereavement outcomes and coping*. Amercian Journal of Men's Health, 15.

shows how we process our deep feelings has not evolved much at all since ancient times.

My personal experience of grief is recent, and presented itself in a form that perhaps is overlooked in the traditional sense of what grieving is.

In 2024, my wife and I suffered two miscarriages. In January 2024, we found out we were expecting a second child. There had been some discussion about if/when we wanted to have child number two before we decided to try again. Shortly afterwards, my wife experienced the typical symptoms of early pregnancy she had had with our first child and a pregnancy test confirmed, much to our surprise, she was pregnant again.

Cue the excitement, nerves, anticipation and everything else that goes with thinking you are going to have a child. We told our parents, started thinking about the future, and decided to go out to dinner to celebrate my wife's birthday. This was 30 January.

As we were getting ready to go out for a delicious meal, my wife called me from the bathroom to say she was bleeding heavily. Though I had never experienced a miscarriage before, my head was immediately there, putting two and two together and assuming she was losing the baby. Despite my own thoughts, I carried on doing my best to reassure my wife it was probably OK and we should not be worried about it. Still, I suggested we went to the hospital just in case.

So, in our restaurant outfits, we drove to the hospital, checked in at the A&E department, were quickly triaged and then went to the onsite GP to be examined.

After waiting for about two hours, we finally spoke to the GP.

Sadly, as with my previous negative experience of GPs, this experience was similar; the male doctor's compassion was limited. He asked how far along we thought she was (at this point it was only about three or four weeks) and asked my wife to take a pregnancy test. The test was negative.

He then talked about how common it was to lose a pregnancy at this stage and just advised taking paracetamol to manage any discomfort. On the journey home, we did not say much to each other, both appreciating the silence. I think we both knew it was not the right time to try to make sense of it all.

After some reflection and expressing of emotion, we agreed that we would just treat it as a false positive rather than a miscarriage. Maybe she was never pregnant? Maybe our test was wrong, and she just had her period as normal? Or maybe we were just tricking ourselves into thinking differently about it.

Probably the last one.

But that worked for us. It was sad (and gutting it had happened on my wife's birthday). Yet the one thing I had not counted on was having to break the news to our parents.

Dealing with your own emotions is one thing; trying to also layer on top the grief and emotions of others adds to the complexity. It is fair to say, my mother loves very hard. By that, I mean she feels her emotions and cares deeply (too deeply) about things and struggles in her own way to process emotions. This often manifests itself in outbursts and lots of overt feelings.

I called her and said what had happened. I explained how we were processing it and were OK, looking to the future rather than dwelling on the past. She was sad for us, upset for the loss, and said what most people say in those situations: "Keep your chin up."

All normal, all fine.

As the days passed, I had more or less parked the event in the far corner of my mind, out of reach of my conscious thoughts and was just thinking about where we would go from there. Periodically I would get messages from my mum, saying how sad I must be and how upset I must feel.

Truth be told, I was sad, but it was not all-consuming; I was upset but was processing it in my own way. In fact, my mum's sorrow made me feel as though I was being pulled back into sadness, making it more difficult for me to move forward.

This was my first real experience of how grief impacts people in different ways, and I learnt that grief is not linear.

Fast forward a month, and we were ready to try again. We waited for another cycle and my wife fell pregnant after our first time of trying. I know that not everyone is as fortunate as this. I have friends who have been trying for years to fall pregnant and some who cannot get pregnant at all. I do not take that lightly.

This time we decided to wait a few more weeks before telling our parents. We also wanted to book ourselves in for an early scan to make sure the pregnancy it was progressing as it should. After about six weeks, no bleeding, all the usual early symptoms – all seemed normal. So, we told our parents again!

We booked ourselves a private scan around eight weeks. Little did I know, the outcome of that appointment would change something in me for ever.

As we waited our turn, we were just chatting as normal, making terrible jokes (that is our way) and feeling fairly positive about the whole thing. Our number was called and in we went. My wife hopped up on the bed, the sonographer confirmed her name, and I took my seat next to her with a perfect view of the screen. Up came a little image and the sonographer confirmed the pregnancy straight away. I smiled a little and sighed with relief that we had not gone mad, and the positive pregnancy test had been correct.

About a minute or so passed and my wife was making her usual awkward small talk when the sonographer interrupted her. Her words made my heart flutter and my breath falter:

"I am so sorry, but there is no heartbeat. I am really sorry I have to tell you, but your baby is not alive."

Silence followed by more silence. Until I broke it with a question. I just needed something to bring me back to the room and also to move us along in the process so we could get out of there. I asked what had to happen next and she told us she would refer us to the hospital and that we had a few options to remove the pregnancy: natural expulsion or surgery.

Either way, the dead baby needed to come out.

We got up, walked out of the building, and my wife started crying. She is not much of a crier but that day I had to support her as we walked to the car. I went straight into 'man' mode, trying to reassure, trying to make it make sense; trying to tell her it was going to be OK and we would get through it.

I just pushed my emotions firmly to the back of my head and locked them away for another day. The miscarriage in January had been early enough to convince ourselves it didn't really happen. But this one?

We had seen the dead baby on the screen – it was as real as it could get.

We made the decision to opt for surgery rather than waiting for nature to take its course. Truthfully, we thought the surgery would be quicker, and we didn't want to experience the physical loss inside our own house.

The problem was we had to wait 10 days for the first available appointment. Those days were wild; such a strange set of emotions, and the odd circumstance of knowing what was inside my wife. Also, just a lot of breath-holding, hoping we made it to the surgery date before her body took control. Fortunately, it did not.

At the hospital was a poster on the wall advertising services for dealing with the grief of baby loss. One of the links was to a government website that allows you to apply for a certificate acknowledging the loss. The purpose is to help bring you closure and to validate that what you had was real and it should not be diminished. While I was waiting for my wife to come out of surgery, I went on the website, filled in the details and ordered the certificate. I had to fill in a box for 'name'. I had no idea what to write so I just put Our Angel (I am not even religious). That felt right at the time, and, in a few weeks, the certificate arrived at the house and has been sitting in a drawer ever since.

Time to tell the grandparents again. Same reactions, same emotions from them. But this time I felt different.

I found myself awake one morning, quite early, pacing up and down in the lounge. Without making it sound too much like a movie, it was dark, raining and the house was deathly quiet.

I could feel the extreme frustration building up in my head slowly turning to anger. I was not angry about what had happened – I was able to reconcile the fact these things do happen and there is nothing we could have done, and it was not our fault. I was angry because I didn't feel I had an outlet for my emotions. As a man, I did not feel comfortable talking about my experience of miscarriage; as a man, I felt I had nowhere to go to talk about a subject so often overlooked from the father's perspective.

One of the key learnings from that experience of grief is this: you need to let it out in some form, ideally a healthy one.

My choice of outlet was by typing it all out on screen. I found it much easier and was much more comfortable putting down in words how I was feeling, as I often struggle to find the right words to verbalise it. Journaling is a recognised way of dealing with complex emotions or traumatic events and that works well for me too. My initial verbal dump was via the professional social network, LinkedIn.

For those who are not familiar with LinkedIn, it is primarily used as a platform to share ideas around business, looking for jobs and building professional networks. Although there are a lot of people in my LinkedIn follower list I know personally, there are thousands whom I have never spoken to, let alone ever met. It felt safer expressing myself on this network to this group of people rather than through something like Facebook, which is made up of my non-work friends. I think this is because my connections on Linked In are professional connections and largely anonymous and there was a sense of safety expressing to that group which I know sounds odd.

There is an evolution on LinkedIn that caught my attention. The overt nature of professional people sharing their personal life stories and experiences has exploded over the past few years. My network is primarily made up of HR professionals as this is what I do for a day job. The altruistic side of these types of posts among this community is about raising awareness and normalising conversations in the workplace.

After posting, and feeling a certain weight lifted from my shoulders and a lightness coming back into my heavy mind, I was not prepared for the response.

Literally thousands of people interacted with my post and shared their own stories, either on the feed of the post itself or by messaging me privately. I had accidentally joined a club that no one really wanted to be in, but it was an active club, nonetheless.

People I had never met or corresponded with before, told me some of their saddest moments in their lives, and thanked me for being brave enough to say it out loud. Such messages came from women as well as men, mothers as well as fathers. Following this overwhelming reaction, something inside me changed. I decided I wanted to use my experiences to try to make positive change in the world, and if anything, good could come from my own trauma, then maybe it would feel like it was meant to be.

That was really the impetus for my wanting to write this book. I had so much built up in my head and I really felt there should be an outlet for men to share their feelings.

How people deal with grief is very personal. Upon reflection, my chosen coping strategy was to set about trying to reframe it and finding a purpose from it. That might not be the same for everyone reading this but finding a positive release for your feelings is a much more sustainable way forward than going down the other route of less positive coping strategies, some of which I will talk about next.

The Mask of Masculinity

For many years, especially in my early 20s, I was told that I was really quite guarded with my feelings and difficult to read. This was said by girlfriends, my mates, my mother, my boss and my colleagues. This was always met with irritation, for my feelings are *my* feelings, what's the problem?

My wife insisted that I go to therapy quite early on in our relationship to talk through my history, my emotions, and why I had those walls built around my true feelings. That is when I first discovered the 'mask of masculinity'.

The 'mask of masculinity' is a concept many psychologists use to describe the emotional barriers men erect in order to maintain an appearance of strength. This façade can become especially pronounced in times of grief, when the rawness of emotion is overwhelming. Men might feel intense sadness, anger, or even confusion, but instead of expressing these feelings, they often bury them under the weight of responsibility or productivity.

Although I was not grieving at the time, the description resonated with me; it was exactly what I did when I felt a certain type of way. I'd just keep myself busy and make myself available to be a good listener to others, believing it would distract me for long enough to forget why I was sad in the first place. I could help other people with their feelings rather than having to acknowledge my own.

A 2010 study entitled *Grieving beyond gender* found that men are less likely than women to openly discuss their grief.[44] This can have serious mental health consequences. The study revealed that men who adhered

---

44 Doka, K.J., & Martin, T.L. (2010). *Grieving beyond gender: Understanding the ways men and women mourn*. Routledge.

more rigidly to traditional masculine norms were at greater risk of prolonged grief disorder (PGD), a condition marked by an inability to heal from a loss over time. These men were also more likely to experience feelings of anger and irritability, sometimes turning to unhealthy coping mechanisms like substance abuse or risky behaviours to deal with their pain.

Has anyone reading this ever distracted themselves through drinking and laughing it off? Yeah, me too.

But we know that responding in this type of way only really has one outcome: masking the real emotional toll, delaying proper mourning and preventing emotional healing.

Grief Is Much More Than Just Emotions

Grief does not only affect the emotional or mental state – it also takes a physical toll on the body. For men, the tendency to suppress emotions can lead to many physical ailments. Studies have shown that unresolved grief can manifest as chronic illnesses, heart problems, and immune system deficiencies. These are all things that we know men naturally suffer more from, without unresolved grief acting as a catalyst.

In one particularly revealing study published in the *American Journal for Public Health*, men who lost their spouses had a significantly higher risk of mortality, particularly from heart disease, in the first year after their loss.[45]

Without being too dramatic, the sentimental reader might liken this to dying from a broken heart.

The phenomenon is known as 'broken heart syndrome' or stress-induced cardiomyopathy (if you prefer the medical version). While it can affect anyone, men are more likely to experience fatal outcomes from heart conditions related to stress and grief. The stress hormones released during grief—namely cortisol and adrenaline—can contribute to heart problems if not properly addressed through emotional release and social support.

It's a Slippery Slope to Suicide

One of the starkest and most tragic outcomes of unresolved grief among men is the elevated risk of suicide. We know that statistically men are three to four times more likely to die by suicide than women, and grief is a significant contributing factor in many cases.

---

45 Kaprio, J., Koskenvuo, M., & Rita, H. (1987). *Mortality after bereavement: A prospective study of 95,647 widowed persons.* American Journal of Public Health, 77, 283-287

The World Health Organisation (WHO) has recognised that men's mental health is often not adequately addressed, despite the alarmingly high rates of depression and suicide linked to grief and loss.

Many men experience a deep sense of isolation in their grief, feeling that they must bear the burden alone. This is exacerbated by societal norms that discourage them from seeking help or expressing their emotions. This combination of emotional suppression, social withdrawal, and the pressure to maintain composure, can be a lethal cocktail, with an outcome that can be fatal.

Breaking the Code of Silence

In recent years, there has been a growing recognition of the need for men to break free from the emotional shackles of traditional masculinity.

Grief counselling and peer support groups that focus specifically on men are increasingly available, providing a safe space for emotional expression. Programs like The ManKind Project and Men's Sheds are designed to encourage men to explore their emotions and seek support without fear of judgement. These efforts are critical in helping men process their grief in a healthy way.

Does it actually work?

Studies suggest that when men are given the tools to express their emotions, their grief can become more manageable. A 2020 study published in the *Journal of Clinical Psychology* found that men who engaged in grief counselling were significantly less likely to experience prolonged grief symptoms and were more likely to maintain better physical and mental health in the long run.[46]

So, in simple terms, there is help available, and by taking the step to seek it out and talk about how you are feeling, you can move through into a more positive place quicker.

Talking Takes Strength – It Is Far from Showing Weakness

Grief is not a weakness, and emotional expression is not a betrayal of masculinity. In fact, one of the strongest acts a man can undertake is to allow himself to feel the full weight of his loss and to seek support in carrying it. The growing body of research on grief in men suggests that the healthiest way forward is through emotional

---

46 Neimeyer, R, Holland, J & Currier, J. (2020). *Meaning reconstruction in the wake of loss*. Journal of Clinical Psychology, 76, 1607-1622.

vulnerability, connection with others, and dismantling the rigid norms that suggest men must always 'keep it together'.

As we collectively become more aware of the specific challenges men face when grieving, I have hope that the cultural narrative will keep shifting. Men will be allowed, even encouraged, to grieve openly, to lean on others, and to prioritise their emotional health.

As I was writing this chapter, the reality show, *I'm a Celebrity Get Me Out of Here*, was being broadcast on UK TV. This show places a group of celebrities into the Australian jungle for three weeks without contact with the outside world.

In one episode, the campmates were getting to know each other a little and started sharing their own stories about trauma in their lives. Famous champion boxer, Barry McGuigan, who was a superstar in the 1980s (and from Northern Ireland like me), told his fellow campmates about losing his daughter to cancer. He talked about how she went from well to ill in a very short space of time and sadly died as a result. Barry, a 'man's man', boxer, tough guy, broke down on various occasions while talking about her. His fellow celebrities crowded round him, gave him hugs and encouraged him to express his emotions.

As I was watching, I thought how terribly sad his story was and such a dreadful loss of life at a young age. But I was so pleased that Barry felt comfortable in his own masculinity to show his real emotions and cry on national television. His campmates remarked how amazing it was to see a man express himself so publicly.

Long may this continue, for this normalising of such emotive male behaviour may not only save lives, but also pave the way for healthier, more emotionally fulfilled men after facing loss.

Grief, though painful and complex, is a deeply human experience. By redefining what it means to be a 'strong' man in the context of loss, we can empower men to honour their emotions and heal from the inside out rather than dying from the outside in.

Showing your emotions does not make you weak; it makes you human.

The following story is from Jack. He is a young man, brother, son and at the time of writing, soon to be husband, who has suffered unimaginable loss in his life. These are his words explaining his own journey with grief.

Jack's Story

As part of GenZ, I would think that it's not unusual for society to have given me a detailed understanding of mental health, whether that be through education, what I view on social media or even the latest viral TV series. However, that was not my experience.

Hello, I'm Jack and I will be sharing a little about my encounters with anxiety and grief. But first, let's rewind.

What I have learnt on my journey of discovery is that so much comes from our childhood. So, what did mine look like? I was really fortunate to have two loving parents and an older brother. While education wasn't a motivator for me, I went to a good state school in the southeast of England. My parents did everything they could to provide for my brother and I – this was to mainly fund our sporting activities and all the accessories that go alongside that. I left school in 2013 and would have described myself as fairly well rounded. The reality was I didn't know anything about real life and that was going to be a steep learning curve.

My first experience of anxiety was playing football as a child. I absolutely loved it and was also quite good as a youngster (that ability has long gone now). By 12, I was playing for two teams and training multiple times a week. When match days came at the weekend, I would be sick and have a panic attack before leaving the house. This was every weekend, without fail. In 2009, no one would have described this as anxiety, but quite simply 'nerves' or, as my parents liked to call it, 'a funny turn'. I started to notice a trend in this behaviour for any big event, or where I felt pressure to perform.

After leaving school and deciding not to pursue full-time education any further, I was determined to start making some money. A few days into my job search, I had an interview as an apprentice with a leading aviation company. Before attending, I vividly remember my dad stopping the car in a nearby service station so I could vomit and have a panic attack. This was seen as normal for me; I was getting worked up and this is how my body eradicated stress. Cut a long story short, I was successful in securing the role and started a career in learning and development, an area I still work in 11 years later.

So, how does grief come into all this? Fast forward to December 2016, I'm working in London, and my role requires me to stay away for multiple nights a week. I return on a Thursday evening and my dad picks me up from the local train station. He gets out of his car and grabs me, crying. Members of the public are looking, and naturally I'm asking what's the matter. My mum that afternoon had decided to take her own life in the family home after a brutal journey with menopause. My whole life changed and has never been the same since.

For the first two years, I decided to ignore any emotion associated with the event and when it was brought up, met the conversation with anger based on her actions, often citing 'selfishness'. I remember only taking two days off work, before returning and keeping myself busy. As a naive 19-year-old, I thought this was effective until one day, after driving two hours into work, I broke down in tears. I was supported by two colleagues, who allowed me to open up in a safe space and supported me. I will always remember that moment.

I quickly utilised the professional services I had available through my employer, and the following week I began attending counselling – something I would have never dreamt of exploring. This naturally brought up a lot of untouched emotion that led to my anxiety ballooning out of control. I would spend days unable to leave the house or even complete a basic task – I was consumed by adrenalin. I had to seek further professional support and reluctantly booked an appointment with my GP. Following a thorough review, I was diagnosed with chronic anxiety and depression; a pretty tough pill to swallow at 21–(if you pardon the pun). Before I knew it, I was trialling a variety of antidepressants, attempting to find the right dosage to balance my hormones. I had so many questions: was I psychotic? Why are the hormones in my brain unbalanced? Was this my mum's fault? Is it hereditary? Will I ever be able to lead a normal life? After what felt like an eternity, I started to stabilise and reacted well to Pregabalin, a controlled class C drug that numbed my adrenal gland, significantly reducing panic attacks, anxiety and overall stress.

However, this wasn't a permanent solution; I was still running away from my emotions. In my spare time I'm a Special Constable and I spent hundreds of hours a month volunteering before and after work, so I didn't have any 'still' moments in my brain. The irony, I was seeing people at their worst, dealing with murders, suicides and violent disorder (just to name a few). For some reason, when I had my uniform on, I was protected from any of my deep-rooted emotions – a means of escapism. Fast forward to 2024, I'm 27 and I'm OK. I have experienced a variety of therapies, from talking to CBT. I have trialled new drugs and attempted to combine and alter over the years; I have changed my diet and the food I eat; I have opened myself up to a level of vulnerability never experienced before. I have embraced my challenges and shared freely to both heal and help support others who may be experiencing similar feelings.

I was in denial for years that anything like this could ever happen to me. The reality... it did. My advice: take that first step. The size will be different for every individual but don't try and battle or take it on yourself. The accessibility of support is better than it's ever been before, so find a pathway that works for you. It's going to feel really low at times, so finding the small wins and those events you seek happiness/reward in is critical. Finally, medication isn't a negative, so with professional support, embrace it and know that with other interventions it will hugely impact your road to full health.

Chapter 8:
Addiction: I Can Stop Anytime

Addiction, while often viewed as an individual struggle, is influenced by a complex set of factors, with gender, especially masculinity, emerging as a significant though often overlooked influence. Across various forms of addiction such as alcohol, drugs, gambling, sex, and pornography, traditional concepts of masculinity shape men's vulnerability, driving patterns of dependence and often blocking paths to recovery. Though I know that men and women can suffer the same effects of addiction, and addiction itself really doesn't know gender boundaries, statistics and studies from the UK, Europe, and globally highlight a distinct pattern: men face higher rates of these addictions, often fuelled by a lot of the things we have talked about in this book: a warped and frankly outdated view of what it means to be a man and masculinity more broadly.

Understanding how masculinity interacts with addiction sheds light on what is yet another silent crisis affecting millions of men; a crisis that requires a deeper rethinking of societal expectations, healthcare approaches, and cultural messages about what it means to be a man.

The Shadow of Addiction in Men's Lives: What do the stats say?

I mentioned about addiction not really caring too much about your gender—alcoholism and drug addiction especially are just as much an issue for women as for men—but the statistics do tell a bit of story about the additional struggle that guys face overall. Let's take a look at what the numbers tell us.

When it comes to addiction, men consistently show higher rates of dependency in certain areas compared to women. Statistics from the UK and Europe certainly highlight these gender disparities, offering a clearer picture of how deeply embedded this issue is across different societies.

- **Alcohol:** Did you know that in the UK, men are nearly twice as likely to experience alcohol dependence as women? Public Health England's 2018 report found that approximately 10% of men aged 16–59 were classified as dependent on alcohol, compared to just 4% of women.[47] For what reason, I hear you ask? Adopting negative coping strategies

---

47 Public Health England. (2018). *Alcohol and Substance Use in the UK: A Gendered Approach*. GOV.UK. Available at https://www.gov.uk/government/publications/delivering-better-oral-health-an-evidence-based-toolkit-for-prevention/chapter-12-alcohol.

such as drinking alcohol is more of a 'man thing'. Often men see drinking heavily as a sign of resilience, camaraderie or dare, I say it, 'fun', particularly in countries with a strong drinking culture.

- **Drugs:** Did you know that men in the UK and Europe are more likely to use and become dependent on illegal drugs? The European Monitoring Centre for Drugs and Drug Addiction (EMCDDA) reports that drug use in Europe is generally more common among men, especially those in their late teens and early 20s.[48] In the UK, the Crime Survey for England and Wales found that around 12% of men aged 16–24 had used a class A drug in the past year, compared to 5% of women in the same age group[49]. Across Europe, men account for approximately 75% of drug-related deaths. That is a huge majority and again support the thought that men tend to engage in more negative coping habits. In this case, it is killing lots of them.

- **Gambling:** Did you know that in the UK, men are four times more likely than women to experience problem gambling? According to 2023 research,

48 EMCDDA. (2022). *European Drug Report 2022: Trends and Developments | www.euda.europa.eu.* Available at: https://www. euda.europa.eu/publications/edr/trends-developments/2022_en.

49 ONS. (2021). *Crime in England and Wales: year ending March 2021 - Office for National Statistics.* Available at: https://www. ons.gov.uk/releases/crimeinenglandandwalesyearending march2021.

Gender and gambling preference, 4.2% of men reported problem gambling, compared to just 1.1% of women.[50] The research also reported that men account for over 80% of participants in high-risk gambling activities such as online sports betting. Across Europe, gambling addiction follows a similar pattern. For example, in Spain and Italy, over 75% of gambling addicts are men, with sports betting seen as both a social activity and a test of 'manliness'. This really should not surprise any of us. Popular sports like football (soccer for our American readers) are littered with adverts for gambling platforms and casinos. It makes me smile, in an uncomfortable way, when they tag the little 'gamble responsibly' line on the end of the umpteenth gambling advert you have seen while waiting for Newcastle to get beaten (yes, I am a Newcastle United fan). There are high profile examples of footballers and other sports professionals who have become gambling addicts, yet guys are often the target audience.

- **Sex and pornography:** Did you know that sexual addiction and problematic pornography consumption also disproportionately affects men? This is one that is perhaps a little less talked about. A UK survey from You Gov in 2022 revealed that nearly 70% of men

---

50 Bacon, P., Conte, A. and Moffatt, P.G. (2023). Gender and gambling preference. *Applied economics*, 56(4), pp.426–439. https://doi.org/10.1080/00036846.2023.2168609.

under the age of 40 view pornography regularly, with one in four men admitting they may be addicted vs only 3% of women.[51] Addiction to porn in particular throws up a lot of issues when it comes not only to the relationships with sex but also the relationship with women when it comes to sex. Porn, by its very nature, gives a distorted reality and it often paints the picture of men dominating women and treating them in a way that is unacceptable. The pressure on men to validate their masculinity through sexual prowess and control feeds into this addiction, with porn often becoming an outlet for unmet emotional, psychological and sexual needs.

Alcohol and Drug Use as 'Proving Grounds'

Being a teenage boy is tricky. It was tricky when I was growing up in the mid-2000s and it is even worse now with societal changes and the emergence of the digital age. Believe it or not, I remember a world without Facebook, X and Instagram, when the only comparisons I really had were the other teenage boys in my immediate peer circle. There was a lot of muddling through and learning together how to become a man. In this pre

---

51 Kirk, I. (2022). *How often do Britons watch porn? | YouGov.* Available at: https://yougov.co.uk/society/articles/42945-how-often-do-britons-watch-porn.

digital world, role models were much more private and less talked about than in today's world. Other than having that one mate who had been through puberty a little quicker and had strong muscles and a terrible beard, there was very little chance of buying booze from a shop without just being laughed at by the people working there.

Back in those days, we would more than likely use our parents or close family as our role models. The world felt much smaller.

My view of alcohol as a teenage boy was one of fear. I very rarely had a drink growing up and that was for the simple reason my mother is an alcoholic. She is a Jekyll and Hyde alcoholic, which for me meant daytime mum was loving, hard-working, caring and fun to be around whereas night-time mum was angry all the time or sad (or both) and impossible to spend time with, so I avoided her whenever I could. My relationship with alcohol was shaped by her relationship with it. I saw firsthand the chaos it caused so it didn't appeal to me.

There is a wonderful Ted Talk from Johann Hari in which he explores addiction through his eyes. He tells us that we think about addiction in completely the wrong way. He says addiction is born out of our need to 'bond' and find connection in the world. There is a story he shares about an experiment on rats in which rats in a cage, with very little else in the cage, were given two options; a normal drink of water and another laced with drugs. In this empty cage, the rats almost always chose the water laced with drugs and almost all of them overdosed every time.

The story and the experiment develop by turning the cage into 'Rat World'. This time, the rats have space to move around, stuff to play on, and interact with each other in a positive social way. They had things to keep them engaged and entertained. Those rats, almost exclusively, drank the non-laced water, and if they did sip on the drugged water, they would do so in moderation and never overdosed.[52]

So, perhaps rather than seeing addiction as a sickness that needs crisis treatment, we need to see addiction as the fallout from a lack of connection people have with others in their lives or a positive environment to flourish in. This interesting twist on how I saw addiction made sense to me, as my own mother only had friends who were drinkers, and she bonded with somehow – perhaps more so than her own family. If I apply this logic to teenage boys growing up and finding their way in the world, then you can see the trouble they might accidentally get themselves into in the quest to bond, especially if they are surrounded by negative influences. This is another argument in favour of prevention rather

---

52 Hari, J. (2015). *Everything You Think You Know about Addiction Is Wrong*. YouTube. Available at: https://www.youtube.com/watch?v=PY9DcIMGxM

than cure. Stopping the addiction taking hold is much easier than treating the addiction once its running rife.

From adolescence onwards, boys often see alcohol and drug use as milestones and rites of passage that prove their worth among peers. Heavy drinking and drug use are frequently romanticised in social settings, leading to an environment where excessive consumption is encouraged as part of being 'one of the guys'. Research published that looks at the links between males drinking and their relationship with masculinity indicates that nearly 40% of young men in the UK see binge drinking as a necessary part of bonding with friends, a statistic that highlights the social expectations that encourage risky behaviour.[53]

One thing I remember is that if one of your mates was from a home where mum and dad were divorced or one of them worked away, then that would be the place to go for the (terrible) house parties.

When I was 16 or 17, I remember going to some house parties with the lads and being the one who would be pretending to drink. I'd have the same Jack Daniels and coke in my hand for hours and never actually swallow any of it. Given the chance, I'd pour some in the plant pot to make it look like I was drinking

---

53 de Visser, R. O., & Smith, J. A. (2007). *Alcohol consumption and masculine identity among young men.* Psychology & Health, 22, 595–614. https://doi.org/10.1080/1476832060094177

it. No one ever said anything. Maybe they were all doing the same thing and it was just a ridiculous masculine game we were all playing without realising it.

However, in my university days, despite my fear of alcohol and personal experiences of watching what it can do to people, I became a categorical binge drinker. This really came about by the need in my mind to fit in. The need to bond overpowered the logic of my lived experiences.

Being a first year at university is all about having fun. Certainly, for me, once I realised that the first-year mark didn't count toward my degree and all I needed to do was pass to come back next year, I made the decision to use university to build life experience rather than academic prowess. I used to get drunk and often went to excessive levels. No sooner had I finished one drink, I would ask where the next one was right away.

For some stupid reason (which to this day I have no idea what made me do it) I made the bold statement in the first drinking session with my new roommates that I only drank Aftershock. For those who do not know what Aftershock is, it is a shot-based drink, tastes absolutely awful, and is a surefire way to make yourself sick if you drink too much of it. The only thing it really has going for it is that it is fairly cheap and also brightly coloured. But in some ridiculous attempt at bravado that became my drink of 'choice' (it really wasn't by choice, more for fear of people thinking I was a loser).

I hated it! Thankfully, a good friend of mine offered me a Bacardi Breezer and thus my relationship with alcopops began and I switched to another brightly coloured drink – WKD Blue. This tasted better and I was thankful not to have to drink shots to prove how 'manly' I was.

When I reflect back on this and compare the younger teenage me, at those house parties pouring Jack Daniels into house plants vs the university me (only separated by a few years) who was drinking awful drinks to try and look cool, I can't help but shudder. What changed in me? The simple truth is my small world growing up suddenly became much bigger and I was thrust into adult life with no safety net. My need to fit in (warped or otherwise) took over and became the dominant thought in my developing mind.

Despite my disdain for alcohol as a child and seeing firsthand the result of alcohol dependence, the desire to 'bond' won the argument in my head. A word of caution for teenagers and young people all around the world: you do not need to get drunk to fit in.

For me, I was always in control (I think), but unfortunately for some, this often spirals into dependency. While I am not saying that every guy who likes a drink builds a dependency, statistically it certainly impacts guys much more than girls.

In fact, according to the Alcohol Health Alliance UK, men are more than twice as likely as women to die from alcohol-related causes.[54] Read into that what you will, but if for teenage boys, they feel the pressure to drink in order to be 'one of the lads; then you can quite easily see how certain behavioural patterns form and habits are created. This is particularly true if alcohol or drugs are being used as a coping mechanism to deal with any of the other topics we have discussed (or will discuss later) in the book.

Joe Gaunt, who we heard from at the beginning of this book, talked to me about the drinking-dopamine cycle. I am no neuroscientist, but I know that dopamine is the happy chemical that is released into our brains when we do something pleasurable. Simple things like walking in the sunshine, eating our favourite foods or exercise are all good examples of our brains sending little signals to our body to say, Yeah, this was fun. So, if we know our body can do this, then what happens if we train our brain to release that dopamine shot when we think about drink or drugs?

Exactly the same thing.

---

54 Alcohol Health Alliance. (2021). *Alcohol Health Alliance responds to ONS figures on alcohol-specific deaths in 2020 - Alcohol Health Alliance*. Available at: https://ahauk.org/news/alcohol-health-alliance-responds-to-ons-figures-on-alcohol-specific-deaths-in-2020/.

We might be visualising Friday coming after a long week at work and picturing that first pint down the pub to welcome in the weekend. Our brains start to create memory circuits and then suddenly every time we think about that same pint at that pub, we start to get happy chemicals before even going. Now we have built an expectation about going to the pub and we crave that happy feeling. That might go on for a while, because having a few drinks at the pub each week isn't bad, is it?

Well, no, there are worse things in the world, but if that Friday drink, then becomes a Saturday drink and maybe a glass or two over dinner every night and perhaps just one more for the road, then it starts to become a problem. Your brain is craving the happy chemicals, and who are you to say no to your brain?

What about when you want to stop?

Our brain does not like that at all. We have built this habit and repetition, so it has now become an expectation. We then try to deny that need. However, human beings are typically wired to have an easy life – we like the path of least resistance. So, if you really want to stop and try to, it will feel uncomfortable for a while as you now have friction of thought and chemicals; you are withdrawing. The simple thing to do would be to have one more drink, that one last taste. You can see how the cycle would just continue and before you even realise it, you are an addict.

If you add to this some of the challenges we have explored, especially about men often being reluctant to ask for help, then the issue is hidden and/or exacerbated through a fear of being seen as weak. This then fuels the addiction even more.

Gambling as a Form of Risk-Taking

Lots of people, men and women, like to gamble – a flutter on the Grand National or the weekly accumulator on the football results. It's perfectly normal and perfectly pleasant to have a flip of a coin on special occasions. When I talk about gambling addiction, I mean those who struggle to think of much else and spend more money than they have to satisfy that thrill or the hope of winning big.

The appeal of gambling taps into a powerful aspect of masculinity: the desire to take risks, prove one's mettle, and claim a sense of control over fate. Gambling in the western world is not only accessible but highly popular among men. I mentioned in the opening of this chapter that football is a popular gambling pastime and advertisers reinforce this. It's common to see at least one gambling advert during a game, whether that be on TV, in the stadium or indeed on the shirts of the biggest teams.

So why do we do it? The buzz and the adrenaline.

Yes, adrenaline, that same chemical we would get from extreme sports like skydiving or being scared in the dark. It makes our hearts beat faster, our muscles feel stronger, and our minds feel sharper.

It is exciting, right?

Sure, of course it is, but this excitement comes with high risks. In the UK, a study by GambleAware revealed that men account for over 75% of the calls to gambling helplines,[55] and they're often seeking help at later stages of addiction, when financial and emotional tolls are already severe.

An article from 2019 that explored the differences between men's and women's health, displayed a model showing three things that typify men.[56] The first, is not seeking help. We have read that a lot in this book. Negative coping is the second part of this model, and things like alcohol and/or drug use fall into this category. The third part of the model is risky behaviour. This is

---

55 GambleAware. (2019). *Annual Statistics from the National Gambling Treatment Service (Great Britain)*.Available at: https:// www.gambleaware.org/our-research/publication-library/articles/ annual-statistics-from-the-national-gambling-treatment-service-great-britain-20192020/ [Accessed 13th November 2024].

56 Harvard Health Publishing (2019). *Mars vs. Venus: The gender gap in health - Harvard Health*. Harvard Health. Available at: https://www.health.harvard.edu/newsletter_article/mars-vs-venus-the-gender-gap-in-health.

firmly where gambling sits – taking risks and putting yourself at risk as a means of distraction or feeling a certain type of way when other things seem to be getting you down. True gambling addicts are chasing that feeling, much like a drug addict or racing car driver is chasing that high.

There are several things that make gambling addiction a real problem to overcome. Firstly, it is difficult to escape the number of gambling adverts and their feeble reminders to 'be gamble aware' and 'when the fun stops, stop'. Alongside this, gamblers can hide their additions easier than other addicts (you could argue that drug addicts and alcoholics have 'tells' in their behaviour that make them a little more obvious, a change in appearance, for example, or a distinct smell on their breath.) But gambling is easier to hide, until it's too late.

The final thing that makes this a particularly troublesome addiction is the ease in which people can do it. Setting up an account on a sports betting app, for example, can be done in a few clicks. These companies have checks and balances in place to confirm identity and have software tools to encourage people to know their limits. But it isn't mandatory or enforced and it is easily ignored. If I was a gambling addict, I would never need to leave my house as I could access multiple different platforms at the click of a button.

Scary, right?

Sex and Pornography as Escapes from Vulnerability

Sex and pornography addiction are especially complex areas, often tied to how men are socialised to view relationships and vulnerability. For many men, intimacy and emotional connection are culturally restricted or scary, leading them to substitute sexual behaviour or pornography as a form of escape or coping mechanism. An article published on the Menshealth.com found 75% of porn is consumed as a way to cope with stress and isolation, while 27% said it helped them 'feel in control' when other areas of their lives felt overwhelming.[57] For lots of people reading this, you might think that watching a bit of porn on your laptop is harmless, and for a lot of people it is. But knowing that people are using it for more than just pleasure i.e. using it as escapism from the troubles of life, puts a different spin on it completely.

I mentioned that gambling is easily accessible, yet by its nature, requires money to participate. Pornography, on the other hand, is even more easily

---

57 Ward, T. (2020). *To Combat Loneliness More Men Are Turning to Porn.* Men's Health. Available at: https://www.menshealth. com/uk/mental-strength/a34640211/men-porn-addiction-male-loneliness/.

accessed and, for the most part, it is completely free of charge.

A quick Google search brings up hundreds of free-to-view porn sites that require no verification or payment. You simply click a button to confirm you are over 18 and away you go. Popular sites like Porn Hub make billions in revenue from users accessing free pornography across increasingly more hardcore categories. It is fair to say there is a genre of porn for everyone. But isn't that scary? No checks or balances, no payment required, and no real way to track what people are watching.

So, why is it a problem, and what are the signs of possible porn addiction?

The biggest issue, amongst men, is the fictional representation of what sex is really like. Porn actors are often chiselled, good-looking guys who are anatomically blessed. They are having simulated sex with good-looking girls who are potentially subjected to increasingly more physical handling than would be acceptable in normal life. Let's discuss a few key themes:

- **Good looks and big packages:** Like we have discussed in the chapter on body image, men are very conscious of their looks and often want what other guys have. Just like on social media, the porn actors portray an unrealistic version of the norm that doubtless causes the guys watching to feel insecure about their own appearance. The difference is that on social media full-frontal nudity isn't commonplace whereas obviously this is encouraged on porn sites. So, picture the scene: you are a guy who is feeling self-conscious about his body. You have a desire to have the six pack and muscular arms you see online. Now you are wondering why you drew the short straw with the size of your penis compared to the guy you were watching on screen. Your self-doubt grows even further. You get into a headspace of loneliness and resentment. And the cycle continues into more negative coping. That is not an unlikely scenario. In fact, I'd say it's something happening all around the world, especially in young men who are trying to find their way with relationships and their own body image. Of course, like the images on social media, what we are seeing in porn is not reflective of reality (for your information, the average erect penis size is somewhere around five and a half inches[58] – not the seven-plus inches displayed by the well-endowed actors.

- **Sex is not really like this:** The categories available for people to watch for free are quite staggering. While these videos feature paid models, they are scripted in a way to simulate things like rape and torture, often

---

58 King, B.M. (2020). *Average-Size Erect Penis: Fiction, Fact, and the Need for Counseling.* Journal of Sex & Marital Therapy, 47(1), pp.80–89. https://doi.org/10.1080/0092623x.2020. 1787279

with the girl being the 'victim'. If you are a guy trying to find your way in the world and perhaps you are feeling like you have no hope of getting a girlfriend, then your perspective on what you need to do to get a girl can be drastically altered by watching this stuff. Just a few clicks of a button on a phone, you can find pornography that shows a guy (or guys) dominating a girl, treating her like a toy and being celebrated for it. If that was my first perception of how sex works, then when it came to the real thing, one of three things would happen: I would either be completely confused. I would feel like real sex is nowhere near as good as the stuff I watch online or there is a real danger of trying to reenact this level of 'torture' on a woman believing it be acceptable. So, the addiction really starts to take hold.

Let us layer on top another key theme of this book: the reluctance of guys to seek help in most situations. Add in a sensitive topic like sex or porn addiction and what do you get? You get silence, shame, hidden and harmful behaviour.

The Centre for Addiction and Mental Health in Canada notes that men often feel intense shame about seeking help for sexual addiction, as it contradicts social expectations about masculinity. This shame can lead to years of struggling in silence, with addiction untreated and reality being continuously distorted.

The Emotional Toll of Addiction on Men

Addiction might well start as a choice but, when it takes hold, it very much becomes a need. Addictive behaviours provide temporary relief or distraction, but they ultimately compound feelings of isolation, guilt and despair. According to the UK's Mental Health Foundation, men with substance dependencies, for example, are three times more likely than not, to report feelings of loneliness, depression and anxiety.[59]

Men's mental health statistics underscore the severity of this hidden crisis. Suicide rates among men in the UK are more than three times higher than for women, with addiction cited as a major factor in many cases. The emotional and social isolation that often accompanies addiction is compounded by a cultural reluctance to embrace vulnerability in men, creating barriers to help. Addiction is used as a coping mechanism and for escapism but if there is no other solution within reach, it is tricky to break the cycle.

Tricky, but not impossible.

The link between masculinity and addiction is entrenched, there is no doubt about that. However,

---

59 Mental Health Foundation (2022). *Men and women: Statistics.* Mental Health Foundation. Available at: https://www. mentalhealth.org.uk/explore-mental-health/statistics/men-women-statistics.

shifts in cultural attitudes, alongside effective support systems, can help break the cycle and redefine masculinity in healthier ways.

Here are some things to think about that could potentially offer a path to changing the narrative on addiction:

- **Encouraging emotional expression:** The fight to normalise vulnerability and emotional expression among men is crucial. Initiatives such as CALM (Campaign Against Living Miserably) in the UK and other mental health organisations have been instrumental in encouraging men to open up about their struggles. Studies show that men who are supported in expressing their emotions are 40% less likely to rely on addictive substances as coping mechanisms.[60] Society must give realistic alternatives to the thing people are addicted to, and that starts by giving people space and permission to feel comfortable talking about it.
- **Promoting healthy relationships and connections:** Isolation is a key factor in addiction. Going back to the view that addiction is a form of bonding, there needs to be healthier things for men to bond over.

---

60 Mental Health Foundation (2022). *Men and women: Statistics*. Mental Health Foundation. Available at: https://www.mentalhealth.org.uk/explore-mental-health/statistics/men-women-statistics.

Initiatives that foster supportive male friendships, such as peer support groups, or activities that encourage connection without substances, have shown significant benefits.[61] This is a powerful argument for things like men's health communities in workplaces – a space for guys to connect, in a positive way, to try to avoid things like addiction and isolation. (Shortly, you are going to read about Matt and how his life changed when he was able to get the support he needed from like-minded people.)

- **Challenging media representations of masculinity:** Media portrayals play a large role in shaping masculinity. Portraying men who prioritise mental health, seek support, and practice self-care can shift norms and encourage a healthier definition of strength. We won't eradicate the porn models or the influencers; we won't eradicate alcohol or drugs, and we won't eradicate gambling sites or sports betting. So, we need to instead change the narrative and help men (especially young men) understand their relationship with these things and connect with realistic stories and imagery, as well as seeking role models who are open about their choices and the path it led them down.

---

61 Prance, K. (2022). *The Importance of Peer Support in Addiction Recovery*. Rehab Recovery. Available at: https://www.rehab-recovery.co.uk/recovery/importance-peer-support-addiction-recovery/.

The following is a story from Matt. He tells a powerful story of addiction and recovery which is truly inspirational. All the words are his own.

Matt's Story

I am a loud, proud gay and sober man nearing 40. I live a happy life in Brighton with a great partner and friends, and full of authentic connections. But this wasn't always the case.

I grew up surrounded by toxic masculinity knowing I was different! I was bullied at school for my sexuality before I really understood it myself and tried hard to blend in and dull my personality. I wasn't one of the boys or girls and felt alone and suicidal. I had thoughts of men in my head and knew I was attracted to them but had no role models or anyone queer in my life is talk to or confide in. I tried to suppress the feelings, thinking they were wrong!

At around the age of 13, I discovered alcohol and later marijuana and ecstasy pills. Getting drunk and high with friends helped me to relax and gave me a false sense of confidence. I found a way to suppress my anxiety and found a love for partying as my way to fit in with my peers.

From early on my drinking led to angry outbursts, blackouts and behaviour that went against my moral compass, but at the beginning I ignored the signs and tried not to care. I grew a thick skin and adopted the attitude of 'I will come for you before you come for me' to protect myself. Yet underneath I was still scared and anxious my sexuality secret would be discovered.

I moved to Brighton and came out. Sleeping with men allowed me to open up that part of my life but it took a few years to really accept love from a man rather than it just being transactional sex.

The drink and the drugs continued through university and beyond. I become a caricature of a loud gay man, full of sexual innuendos, drinking to the point of blackout and having sex with anyone who would pay me attention. I would fall in love and cheat, lose jobs, fall out with friends and family – my life was a hurricane of drama.

My mental health deteriorated, and the blackouts got worse. I would have run-ins with the police, waking up with various unexplained injuries and get involved in abusive relationships. I was no longer having fun but couldn't stop the cycle. I would live in fear of what drunk me had said and done, and the only way to ease the shame was to drink again which led to further drama. I became involved in the 'chemical sex' scene and the drugs got harder, leading to sleep deprivation, psychosis, sexual diseases, and losing a grip on reality. With apps, anonymous sex was too easy.

I tried therapy, smart recovery and changing drinks and patterns to try to stop drinking but nothing worked. I spent five years on the brink of suicide knowing that life wasn't working, and I had no purpose but was unable to stop drinking. I would wear a mask to make others think I was living the party lifestyle, but I was broken inside.

I considered rehab and decided as a last-ditch attempt to try a 12-step meeting. I eventually found a group of people who had the same anxieties, thoughts and powerlessness over alcohol that I had, and I was able to start my sobriety journey.

Five years have now passed. I understand some of us have a reaction to alcohol that means we obsess over it and can't stop once we put the first drink inside us and that leads to the Jekyll and Hyde behaviour. As time went on, I was able to peel back my defence layers and unpick the drunk sexual character I had created to protect the scared boy within.

Gaining self-esteem enabled me to learn to value and care for myself, to recognise my gifts and shine them bright. Not everyone needs to understand or like me, but I try to put positive energy out in the world.

The voices in my head and the negative self-talk are not real, and over time you can learn to treat yourself with love and compassion. Talk to people about what goes on in your head – don't bottle things up. I now try my best each day to see the positives in life, be grateful for what I have, try to look at things from other perspectives, and know I'm not perfect but try my best and that's OK. I try to help others and encourage you to do the same and know that mental health can go up and down but make the best of life when you feel good.

There was so much shame in my life, firstly around my sexuality then over my drunken behaviour. But I am now proud to call myself gay and an alcoholic because I own my past, and these are now strengths I can use to help others struggling.

I hope that as time evolves, people will have less stigma attached to sexuality but think it can still be difficult to come to terms with being different in a straight world! Look for support from those who have come out before you. I love my life as a gay man now and wouldn't have it any other way.

If you are questioning your relationship with alcohol or drugs, then don't wait until it gets really bad! There are great support services out there and I would recommend 12-step support groups. Don't suffer in silence. It will feel like you can't imagine a life without substances, but I promise life is so much better sober! It's not easy but once you discover your true self and passion for life it makes all that hurt worth it.

Learn to love yourself; everything is as it's meant to be. Build others up and practice love, tolerance, patience and understanding. Life begins at sober…

Chapter 9:
Where Do We Go from Here?

Throughout this book I have tried to peel back a layer or two to reveal the struggles that men and boys have in this current version of our world. My idea of writing all this down, digging into research and telling real stories, was to show that the future of our world needs men to feel and operate at their very best, and it is important for the advancement of the equality campaign that men are part of the conversation.

I have uncovered shocking statistics and lived experiences about what it is really like to be a guy. I have explored topics that now seem to be getting attention like men's physical and mental health and suicide rates, while also shining a light on other areas that could be considered historically taboo. Things like domestic abuse, body image and addiction are not openly discussed despite having a profound impact on men and boys.

But like any good storytelling, we need a solid ending. I am fortunate enough to attend and speak at many events, and I always provide a summary and give the audience some practical next steps to take away.

This is all done with the aim of sparking a conversation and curiosity to do things differently.

These are my top strategies for you to consider that may just make that difference to you or the men in your life.

Find Your Purpose and Be Comfortable with your Identity

Every man's journey to identity and purpose is unique, but it is a journey worth undertaking. The stakes are high – without a clear sense of who you are and why you exist, life can feel hollow and overwhelming. Conversely, with a strong identity and compelling purpose, you can navigate life's challenges with confidence, resilience and fulfilment.

Remember, the process of discovering your identity and purpose is ongoing. It requires introspection, action and the courage to face uncomfortable truths. Start today by asking yourself:

- Who am I when no one is watching?
- What gets me out of bed in the morning?
- How can I use my strengths to serve others?

We crave changes in society, and more policy support and resources for men's mental and physical health is absolutely vital if we want to turn the tide of the crisis, we are currently in. But do not lose sight of the part that men play in their own health. We must take more accountability for our feelings, decisions and emotions, and a big part of that is taking some time to reflect on who we are and why we are here. There is no doubt in my mind that every man on this planet can and should have a positive impact on their world, however big or small it is for them. It must start with reflection to build self-awareness.

Whatever the historic or current view of masculinity, you should be comfortable with who you are. Knowing what you stand for, and your strengths and your weaknesses softens the need to compare yourself to others or believe you need to act in a certain way just to portray what you think a man is. The answers to these simple questions can transform your life. As you clarify your identity and align it with your purpose, you will not only improve your own wellbeing but also inspire and uplift those around you.

The biggest superpower men can have is knowing their own self-worth and that being enough for them.

Create the Space for Meaningful Connections and Keep Them Warm

Feeling lonely in the 21st century really should not be a thing—we are so connected in our digital world of eight billion people—but yet we can feel isolated and on our own. We know from the statistics and personal stories in this book that men are more likely to experience loneliness than women, and this is particularly true in early adulthood and later life. As guys, we owe it to each other to be the friend we would want to have. If you are one of those people who has lost touch with a friend or a group of mates and you keep meaning to give them a call or shoot them a text, do it now. The research is clear: we are community-based creatures, and isolation kills.

Remember, there is a difference between being alone and being lonely. Creating spaces where men can interact and connect with each other in an authentic way is a crucial cog in the machine to help us battle the loneliness pandemic. Men are more likely to feel comfortable in settings where connection is not the sole focus of the conversation. This is why things like sports and community groups that have a particular likeminded interest work well, because guys can bond over the love of the thing, they are there to participate in without feeling the awkwardness of trying to make new friends.

The value of friendship and bonding should be taught from an early age. Helping and encouraging children to have friends and see the importance of being around other human beings, especially during teenage years, is a game changer. Teenagers are going to seek connection somewhere, it is human nature, so, we must ensure that such connections are healthy rather than people being pulled into polarised groups who only seek to divide.

Barriers to groups which focus on men's health topics and connection are not dangerous to equality. In fact, they are vital to furthering the equality march. There are things that directly impact men more than women and a lack of meaningful relationships is one of those things. This is particularly true of the workplace. Remember, one in four people experience frequent loneliness in the workplace and two thirds of people do not feel a sense of belonging. Lots of work has been done to create ERGs for unrepresented parts of society in recent years that focus on education and allyship.

Men need to be included in these ERGs, not as an unrepresented group (men are not unrepresented in wider society) but rather as a community that provides a safe space for men to discuss their lives, educate themselves on male-specific issues, and understand the importance of being a positive ally to the other groups (especially any women's networks). There is a nervousness from many businesses to do this, but I am pleased to say that there are a lot more organisations waking up to the fact guys have guy troubles, and they need to have a space in which to feel connected.

As we approach later life, we must not forget the elderly, especially elderly men. Sadly, as we get older the feelings of isolation are magnified as people around us drift or pass away. Making sure we check in on our older friends or neighbours, even if it's just to have a cup of tea or a quick chat, can make a huge difference to their physical and emotional health. Knowing that you matter to someone is a lifeline when people are feeling at their very worst.

Be the Ally the World Needs

In an increasingly hostile world, men have a key role to play in bringing some kindness and empathy. While these traits might be naturally more feminine in nature, guys should work to build these skills to enable fruitful relationships and interactions to develop.

There is no doubt that the actions of men in history have created some disdain and fear – we should not be living in a world where women do not feel safe to walk home at night or are worried about dressing a certain way in case they attract unwanted attention. But not all guys are predators. In fact, most men reading this will be horrified by the actions of their fellow males. But this is not the time to have the attitude of 'I'd never do that' as it simply dismisses the concerns of women and girls in our world.

The facts are the facts: men are much more likely to be perpetrators of domestic abuse; men are much more likely to be perpetrators of sexual assault or rape, and men are much more likely to be violent. Understanding the facts and having an awareness and empathy of how this can impact the women and girls in your life, is a good place to start.

But it is not enough.

Are you the ally that the world needs? Men should be making more effort to champion the inclusion debate; men should be making more effort to support events like International Women's Day; men should be educated on issues that impact women, like the menopause. Knowledge is power, and if we can combine that with an effort to increase our empathy and kindness, then we can help to make the world a better place.

If you are a guy still thinking, *Yeah, but that is not me*, then try thinking of this call to action like this: if you are kind, empathetic, supportive of women's issues and modern in your mindset, then you have the biggest role of all.

Too many bad men get the attention because not enough good men stand up to say no.

Do not be a bystander if you witness poor behaviour in your family or friendship groups; call out so-called 'banter' that crosses the line into sexual harassment. Showcase *your* version of masculinity to others so the good men can dominate the narrative, and the bad men can disappear into insignificance.

Find the People that Make you Feel Good About Yourself

If the saying about being a product of your environment is true, and your environment is negative, then it is time to change it. By this I mean we need to do more to understand the importance of the people around us and, specifically, the people we look up to – our role models.

There are two things to think about. Firstly, who are the role models in your life? If you are one of the many men who spends time comparing himself to unrealistic models online or in the public eye, then consider the impact that is having on your behaviour and self-esteem. Although it is natural for us to compare ourselves to other men and think how we want what another guy has (good looks, money, girls, cars, careers), we also have control over what we view as real.

Of course, it's often easier said than done, but taking back the control of your own emotions and feelings is a powerful thing. Find role models whom you admire and value because of their principles and beliefs rather than their looks and money; follow people who speak openly about their emotions rather than those who make light of feelings and tell you to 'man up'. If you are in a friendship group in which you feel unable to be authentic, then it might be time to consider whether being in that friendship group is worth it. Surrounding yourself with people who make you feel positive about yourself, in a healthy way, is a choice.

Role models do not need to be influencers or politicians. They can be friends, parents, uncles, brothers and colleagues. Role models can also be you.

Now for the other side of the coin: what type of role model are you? What influence are you having on those around you? Are you positively shaping the future generation of guys?

Actions have consequences, and how you behave and interact is noticed. If you are concerned that your son, nephew, brother or friend is being influenced in a negative way, then are you doing enough to show them another path?

Educating young men in relationships, manners, online safety, the dangers of disinformation, and the importance of things like consent, is crucial to help us build a future generation of productive and kind guys. Also, show them that it is OK to be vulnerable and that talking about feelings is encouraged. Young men will look to those around them to help shape their own identity. If they see you as a person who values conversations, loves connection, has healthy coping habits, talks about feelings, takes care of himself physically and mentally, and normalises conversations around things like sex and mental health, then you will be a positive influence and will help shape him to be the same.

Practice your Positive Coping

When times are tough and the pressure is on, men are more likely than women to partake in negative coping strategies such as substance abuse, taking unnecessary risks and pleading ignorance.

The relationship that men have with their feelings is complicated, and we should recognise this when trying to devise ways to help. In my experience of wellbeing, especially through the police and in the corporate world, much of the time, the effort and money go into crisis support. I completely understand why this happens – the crisis stuff is scary and memorable; it is the stuff that hits the headlines and leaves a lasting impression. Of course, we need to have more resources in place to help the growing need for crisis intervention more broadly in the space of mental health. However, the untapped area of wellbeing, and in this case about helping men cope, is about making a more concerted effort in the prevention space.

We need to put more emphasis on prevention rather than cure; we need to encourage the seeking of medical help before it becomes fatal; we need to stop addiction before it takes hold, and we need to stop suicide before it is too late.

How do we do it? Policy, law and government intervention are all important. I was delighted to read the recent announcement by the UK's Health and Social

Care Secretary that the government intends to develop the first ever men's health strategy. Although in its early stages, this massive step forward will aim to put a plan in place to tackle things that are affecting men of all ages and costing lives needlessly. It flags things like heart disease and, prostate and testicular cancer, as well as mental health and suicide prevention.

The fact that the UK Government is acknowledging the need for direct intervention, is really positive. I will certainly be watching carefully to see what progress is made. We should not shy away from the fact that men are disproportionately affected by certain things and should celebrate the fact that if we can help men to live happier, longer and healthier lives, then the impact will not only be felt by them, but all those males and females with which they come into contact.

When it comes to the details and how prevention rather than cure can become a reality, policy can only play a small part. The other crucial part is that men need to take assertive action for themselves. We need to normalise things like medical checks if something doesn't feel right in our testicles; we need to get our prostates checked if we have any concerns; we need to seek medical intervention if we are feeling unwell and take the medication prescribed. Whatever level of embarrassment or shame we may experience when seeing a GP, this is nothing compared to the pain and suffering that will come by ignoring it.

If you are stressed and not sure where to turn, try speaking to someone you trust or seek professional help, rather than going it alone or adopting negative coping strategies. Positive coping is about being consciously aware of how you are feeling and learning how to handle that emotion. If the answer is to pick up a beer or smoke some weed every time you feel a certain way, then recognising that, acknowledging it and trying to change that behaviour is crucial. No addict in the world sets out to be an addict, it happens before you know it. Do not be that guy.

Be aware of your nutrition, sleep patterns and physical activity. Creating a positive relationship with food, exercise and sleep will help build resilience when times are tough. If you are reading this and thinking you want to make a change, remember that forming new habits can be tough at first, and it takes time and effort, so don't get demoralised. Knowing it'll be hard but sticking with it and seeing it through to the end is a great way to take back control.

Conclusion

I set out to write a book that shone a light on the notion of masculinity and why men are struggling in the modern world. I wanted to also highlight the things men think about and worry about and how our relationships with the world can be complex.

Men, and young men more specifically, are feeling a sense of identity crisis. In just a generation, the meaning of what it means to be a man has been detonated by the quick march of equality. We are seeing young men growing resentful as they struggle to see themselves in the media representation of a man and are frightened to speak about how they feel for fear of not being taken seriously or being told they are privileged and should be grateful.

This confusion is magnified by terms like toxic and positive masculinity. At the beginning of the book I talked about the two forms of masculinity offered to men: option A and option B:

Option A: Positive masculinity. On the face of it, this sounds great. The traits of this option include things like kindness, empathy and emotional expression but a confused young man may interpret this as being less like a man and more like a woman as these traits are naturally and traditionally more associated with females.

Option B: Conservative masculinity. These are traits that encourage men to be dominant, the strong one, treat women disrespectfully, and to take back control. When this option is glamorised by famous faces and politicians, we can see why many confused young men see the appeal of option B over option A.

My ultimate call to action is to develop an option C – where men can develop positive skills and build their self-awareness, as well as recognising there are things that impact us more than women and that we need to talk about them openly.

We are running the risk of polarising a whole generation of young men and leaving them behind. We know the statistics on men's mental and physical health, and we understand the concern around education standards. So, now we need to act before they become a lost generation.

Whether you are a man reading this in your later years, a young man trying to build some knowledge to help you work out what to do next, a mother concerned about the future of her son, or a business leader wondering if you should take the leap and support men in your organisation, there is lots going on behind the I'm fine exterior. Putting these actions into play and acknowledging the themes in this book are real is an amazing start.

If we all work together to raise awareness of men's mental and physical health, take accountability for our actions, and show genuine care for all parts of our community, then we can reset society's view of masculinity and create a balanced and healthy world for everyone.

Men's Health Support

https://uk.movember.com/about/foundation
www.bhf.org.uk
www.nhs.uk
www.samaritans.org
www.mind.org.uk
www.cancerresearchuk.org
www.unifymen.com
www.mankindprojectuki.org
www.menshealthforum.org.uk
www.mensadviceline.org.uk
www.nationaldahelpline.org.uk
https://mankind.org.uk/

www.ingramcontent.com/pod-product-compliance
Ingram Content Group UK Ltd.
Pitfield, Milton Keynes, MK11 3LW, UK
UKHW040018160725
6910UKWH00001B/4